Renewing Items
When Renewing Items Please Make Sure You Have Your Library Card With You

You Can Renew By:

Sandwell Library
External: 0121 507 3587
Internal: 3587
Email: swb-tr.ClinicalLibrary@nhs.net
Online: www.base-library.nhs.uk

City Library
External: 0121 507 5245
Internal 4491
Email: swb-tr.BevanLibrary@nhs.net
Fines apply see library notice boards

before the last d   vn below

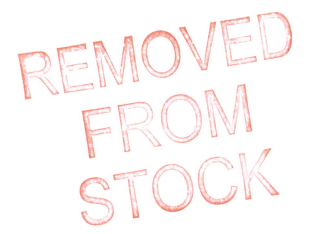

Examination Techniques in Orthopaedics

Second Edition

Examination Techniques in Orthopaedics

Second Edition

Edited by

Nick Harris FRCS (Tr&Orth)

Consultant Orthopaedic Surgeon, Department of Orthopaedic Surgery, Leeds General Infirmary,
Leeds, UK

Fazal Ali FRCS (Tr&Orth)

Consultant Orthopaedic Surgeon, Department of Orthopaedics & Trauma, Chesterfield Royal
Hospital, Chesterfield, UK

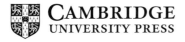

CAMBRIDGE
UNIVERSITY PRESS

CAMBRIDGE
UNIVERSITY PRESS

University Printing House, Cambridge CB2 8BS, United Kingdom

Published in the United States of America by Cambridge University Press,
New York

Cambridge University Press is part of the University of Cambridge.

It furthers the University's mission by disseminating knowledge in the
pursuit of education, learning and research at the highest international levels
of excellence.

www.cambridge.org
Information on this title: www.cambridge.org/9781107623736

© Cambridge University Press 2014

Second edition first published 2014
First edition first published 2003

Printed in the United Kingdom by TJ International Ltd. Padstow Cornwall

A catalogue record for this publication is available from the British Library

Library of Congress Cataloguing in Publication data
Advanced examination techniques in orthopaedics.
Examination techniques in orthopaedics / edited by Nick Harris, Fazal Ali. –
Second edition.
      p. ; cm.
Preceded by: Advanced examination techniques in orthopaedics / edited by
Nick Harris ; assistant editor, David Stanley. 2003.
Includes bibliographical references and index.
ISBN 978-1-107-62373-6 (Hardback)
I. Harris, Nick, 1965-editor of compilation.   II. Ali, Fazal, 1962-editor of
compilation.   III. Title.
[DNLM: 1. Musculoskeletal Diseases–diagnosis.   2. Orthopedic
Procedures–methods.   3. Musculoskeletal Abnormalities–diagnosis.
4. Musculoskeletal System–injuries.   5. Physical Examination–methods.
WE 141]
RC925.7
616.7′075–dc23   2013025681

ISBN 978-1-107-62373-6 Hardback

To Becky, Lucy, Rosie, Molly, Jack and not forgetting Nelson and Henry. A great team.

To Gill, Reza and Sara. For the years of loving support and encouragement without which my contribution would not be possible.

Contents

Contributors

Amjid Ali FRCS (Tr&Orth)
Consultant Shoulder and Elbow Surgeon,
Sheffield Teaching Hospitals NHS Foundation Trust,
Sheffield, UK

Fazal Ali FRCS (Tr&Orth)
Consultant Orthopaedic Surgeon, Chesterfield Royal
Hospital, Chesterfield, UK

L. Chris Bainbridge FRCS
Consultant Orthopaedic Hand Surgeon,
Royal Derby Hospital, Derby, UK

Derek Bickerstaff MD, FRCS, FRCSEd
Consultant Orthopaedic Surgeon,
One Health Group, Sheffield, UK

Stephen Bostock FRCS (Orth)
Consultant Orthopaedic Hand Surgeon,
Sheffield Teaching Hospitals NHS Foundation Trust,
Sheffield, UK

Neil Chiverton FRCS (Tr&Orth)
Consultant Orthopaedic Spinal Surgeon,
Northern General Hospital, Sheffield, UK

Ashley Cole FRCS (Tr&Orth)
Consultant Orthopaedic Spine Surgeon,
Sheffield Children's Hospital, Sheffield, UK

Alexandra Dimitrakopoulou MD
Hip Fellow, Spire Cambridge Lea Hospital,
Cambridge, UK

James A. Fernandes FRCS (Tr&Orth)
Consultant Orthopaedic Surgeon, Sheffield Children's
NHS Trust and Barnsley District General Hospital, UK

Joe A. Garcia FRCS (Tr&Orth)
Consultant Hand Surgeon, Chesterfield Royal
Hospital, Chesterfield, UK

Nick Harris FRCS (Tr&Orth)
Consultant Orthopaedic Surgeon, Leeds General
Infirmary, Leeds, UK

Stanley Jones FRCS (Tr&Orth)
Consultant Orthopaedic Surgeon, Sheffield Children's
Hospital, Sheffield, UK

Simon Kay FRCS (Plas)
Professor of Plastic Surgery, Leeds Teaching Hospitals
NHS Foundation Trust, Leeds, UK

David Limb BSc, FRCS (Orth)
Consultant in Trauma and Orthopaedic Surgery,
Leeds Teaching Hospitals NHS Foundation Trust,
Leeds, UK

Peter Millner FRCS
Consultant Spinal Surgeon, Leeds General Infirmary,
Leeds, UK

Tom Smith FRCS, FRCSE
Emeritus Orthopaedic Surgeon, Sheffield Teaching
Hospitals NHS Foundation Trust, Sheffield, UK

David Stanley FRCS
Consultant Orthopaedic Surgeon, Sheffield Teaching
Hospitals NHS Foundation Trust, Sheffield, UK

Ian Stockley FRCS
Professor of Orthopaedics, Sheffield Teaching
Hospitals NHS Foundation Trust, Sheffield, UK

Richard Villar FRCS
Consultant Orthopaedic Surgeon, Spire Cambridge
Lea Hospital, Cambridge, UK

Robert Winterton MPhil FRCS (Plast)
Hand Fellow, Leeds Teaching Hospitals NHS Trust,
Leeds, UK

John E. D. Wright FRCS (Tr&Orth)
Consultant Orthopaedic Upper Limb Surgeon,
Chesterfield Royal Hospital, Chesterfield, UK

Foreword

I am pleased to be asked to write the foreword for the second edition of *Examination Techniques in Orthopaedics*, coedited by Mr Nick Harris and Mr Fazal Ali. The first edition of this textbook was one of the bestselling orthopaedic books in the United Kingdom for almost a decade. This second edition is likely to at least equal that success. So often in the world of orthopaedic surgery we jump to advanced imaging and forget about the importance of the examination. This is clearly a mistake and has caused many errors in clinical judgement. Therefore, careful review of orthopaedic examination as presented in this textbook is critical for all orthopaedic surgeons, young and old alike. This book provides a complete repository of all examinations, beginning with general principles and proceeding literally from head to toe, to include paediatric examination. This is truly an excellent book and likely will be the gold standard to which examination textbooks are compared. It is my pleasure to write this foreword. I think you will enjoy this textbook and it should stay on your shelf until the third edition is available. I give it my strongest endorsement and look forward to studying it myself.

Mark D. Miller, MD
S. Ward Cassells Professor of Orthopaedic Surgery
Division Head, Sports Medicine
Team Physician, James Madison University
JBJS Deputy Editor for Sports Medicine
Director, Miller Review Course
Charlottesville, VA, USA

Preface

The first edition of this book has become essential reading for those preparing for postgraduate examinations in orthopaedics. Medical students and junior trainees had their own books to use. This is surprising as the same process of examination is used by all groups, the only differences being that the senior trainee should look more polished and should know more special tests. It was this realization that prompted us to come together with our many years' experience of teaching clinical examination and to rewrite every chapter in a format that was uniform in style and in a sequence that could be used in examination situations or in clinical practice by all. Quick revision will become easier as each chapter ends with a summary of the examination technique. Another unique addition is that the illustrations also follow a sequence for quick visual revision. These illustrations are supplemented by numerous new clinical photographs. It is our hope that we have made this book even more user-friendly and an essential companion through your career in clinical practice.

Fazal Ali and
Nick Harris

Acknowledgements

This edition would not have been possible without the help of many. Paul Banaszkiewicz and Nicholas Dunton from Cambridge University Press came up with the idea of combining the first edition with the manual from the Chesterfield FRCS(Tr&Orth) clinical course. Joanna Chamberlin took over as Medical Editor at Cambridge and guided us through the production of this edition.

We are especially grateful to the Yorkshire Foot and Ankle Group for their Educational Grant and Biomet for their continuing support of medical education.

We are grateful for the help from Karsten Edwards at IMM models, and Nicole and Ami our models, who have done their best to inspire another generation of orthopaedic surgeons. Thank you to Oghofori Obakponovwe, orthopaedic trainee, for being the male model in many of the photographs!

Thanks to Nigal Oram, medical photographer for many of the clinical photographs and not to forget the patients who consented to be photographed especially Philip Wagstaff who insisted he pose for the brachial plexus chapter!

Thank you to our own teachers of clinical examination including Mike Bell, John Getty, Tom Smith, Ian Stockley, David Stanley and Colin Beauchamp. To our colleagues in training that helped to mould us in preparation for our own exams especially James Fernandes, Irwin Lasrado, James Williams and Shantanu Shahane. And, last but not least, the many medical students and orthopaedic registrars whom we taught over the years and who allowed us to perfect the art of clinical examination in order to write this second edition.

Nick Harris and
Fazal Ali

General principles of orthopaedic clinical examination

Stanley Jones and Fazal Ali

Clinical examination is an art and has to be learnt, as it does not come naturally. All patients must be respected, made to feel at ease and assured of their confidentiality and dignity.

A detailed history should always be taken followed by clinical examination.

It is often assumed that clinical examination begins on the couch. This should not be the case, as significant information can be gained by observing the patient as they enter the room and walk towards you or as you approach them.

If the patient is seated they should be asked to stand as this is usually the first part of any orthopaedic clinical examination, except when the hand is being examined. You will observe whether the patient is tall, short, fat, thin, ill, well, energetic or slow. Observe if there is pain or if there are stigmata of orthopaedic disease such as blue sclera (osteogenesis imperfecta), café-au-lait spots (neurofibromatosis), multiple exostoses (diaphyseal aclasis; Figure 1.1), etc.

In addition, the gait pattern, any limb deformities and the use of walking aids will also be noted. This is particularly relevant when examining the lower limbs and spine.

Examples of gait patterns include:

- antalgic gait caused by pain that could be from the sole of the foot to the hip. The stance phase of the affected limb is shortened;
- high stepping gait is seen in patients with hereditary sensorimotor neuropathy or those with a foot drop.

The clinical signs and associated deformities of some clinical conditions, e.g. hallux valgus, may be so characteristic that the diagnosis can be made without a full clinical examination. However, this is not always the case, and an examination carried out in a systematic manner not only instils confidence in the patient but avoids missing important and salient clinical signs.

The system of **look, feel, move** advocated by Apley is what we recommend, although when examining the wrist and elbow **look, move, feel** may be preferred.

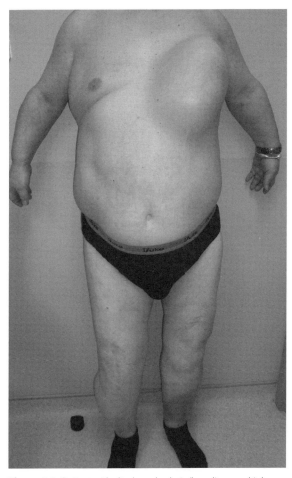

Figure 1.1 Patient with diaphyseal aclasis (hereditary multiple exostoses). Note the short limbs, bowing of the forearm, swellings around the knees and the large tumor in the left pectoral region.

Examination Techniques in Orthopaedics, Second Edition, ed. Nick Harris and Fazal Ali. Published by Cambridge University Press. © Cambridge University Press 2014.

The part of the musculoskeletal system being examined must be suitably exposed; for example, when examining the shoulder the patient should be undressed to the waist. Modesty in females should be preserved by using a strapless garment to cover the breasts. The patient must be given clear instructions on which clothes to take off. The ease or difficulty of undressing and any associated pain experienced whilst doing so is useful information that helps in the assessment. In addition, it is advisable to expose both limbs for comparison even though only one limb may be affected.

Examination of paediatric patients requires skill and flexibility. Remember to look at the parents as the patient may be presenting with an inherited clinical condition. More information can be acquired by adopting methods of play than using a rigid system of examination as previously suggested. Any tests for tenderness must be carried out at the end.

Equipment

The basic equipment required for orthopaedic examination includes a tape measure, goniometer and tendon hammer. In addition to these tools, a pen, key and coin are required for assessment of hand function (Figure 1.2).

Look

Inspection is the initial part of any examination and should always be undertaken before palpation and movement. It also forms an important part of palpation and movement.

It is important to look at the part being examined from various angles, e.g. the shoulder joint should be observed from the front, back and side and the axilla must also be inspected. Inspection of the foot is not complete without examining the sole and between the toes. Whilst observing a limb any scars, skin colour changes, swelling, bruising, muscle wasting or alteration in shape or posture are noted. Scars may be the result of injury or previous surgery. Skin colour changes may be the results of infection, vascular compromise or pain syndrome.

Swelling may be localized or diffuse. Localized swelling and its location with respect to the underlying anatomical structures usually gives a clue as to the possible cause, e.g. a well defined swelling in the radiovolar aspect of a wrist is likely to be a ganglion. A swelling on the medial joint line of the knee is likely to be a meniscal cyst.

Diffuse swelling confined to a joint may be the result of excessive:

- synovial fluid from an inflammatory process such as rheumatoid arthritis or osteoarthritis;

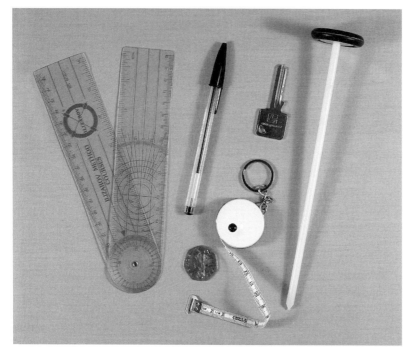

Figure 1.2 Equipment required for examination.

- blood (haemarthrosis) from a recent injury, blood coagulation defect or medication such as warfarin;
- pus from an infection.

Bruising is usually the result of trauma to tissues owing to a recent injury or surgery. Muscle wasting may arise from disuse because of pain, other abnormality or muscle denervation. Muscle wasting is quantified by comparing the affected limb with the normal limb or by measuring the circumference of the limb at a fixed point from a bony landmark.

Alteration in shape or posture may be caused by a congenital anomaly, skeletal dysplasia, joint degeneration or the sequelae of a previous injury.

Finally, inspection should involve looking for and describing any orthosis or walking aid.

Inspection should always be thorough. In clinical examinations at a junior level it is desirable to describe both positive and negative findings. In more senior examinations inspection should still be complete, but is performed much more rapidly with only positive and important negative findings expressed. Examiners may become agitated if senior candidates spend too much time on inspection.

Feel

Irrespective of the joint being examined palpation should always be carried out in a systematic manner with reference to the anatomic landmarks. The details of how to carry out a satisfactory palpation of the various joints are discussed in the relevant chapters, but an essential aspect of palpation is that the examiner must not only look at the joint being examined but also look at the patient's face to appreciate any areas of tenderness (Figure 1.3).

Ensure that hands are washed or antiseptic gel is used. Rubbing your hands together to warm them makes palpation more comfortable.

Some joints, such as the hip and shoulder, are deeper and therefore significant information may not be gained by palpation compared to the more superficial joints such as the hand, elbow, spine, knee, foot and ankle. By knowing the surface anatomy of these joints, tenderness over the relevant areas may lead to the diagnosis, e.g. tenderness over the lateral epicondyle of the elbow indicates tennis elbow and tenderness over the medial joint line of the knee may indicate a medial meniscus tear.

Move

Both active and passive range of movement of the joint being examined should be assessed. It is advisable to carry out active range of movement before passive as this gives the examiner an idea of the functional range of movement and any associated pain. The patient must be given clear instruction or a demonstration of the range of movement to be carried out. Demonstration is sometimes the best method of communicating to the patient.

- It is always advisable to compare the range of movement of the symptomatic with the asymptomatic or normal joint, and the range achieved should be recorded in degrees as measured by a goniometer.
- Sometimes it may not be possible to assess active range of movement in certain situations (such as with a very young child or a patient with cerebral palsy or other neurological disorder).

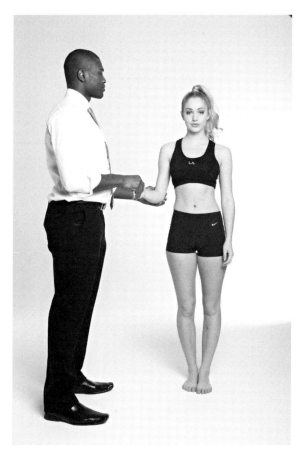

Figure 1.3 Observe the patient closely whilst examining.

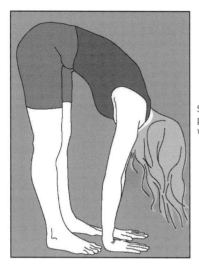

Score one point if you bend and place your hands flat on the floor without bending your knees

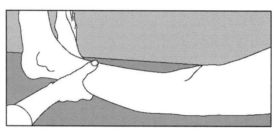

Score one point for each knee that hyperextends

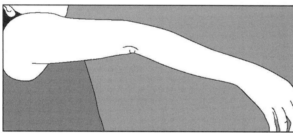

Score one point for each elbow that hyperextends

Score one point for each thumb that will bend back backwards to touch the forearm

Score one point for each hand when you can bend the little finger MCP joint back beyond 90°

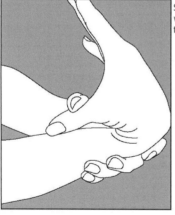

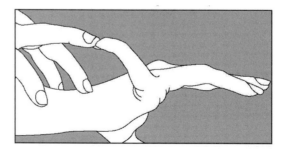

If you are able to perform all of the above manoeuvres you have a maximum score of 9.

Figure 1.4 Beighton's score.

- Complete loss of (active and passive) movement may be the result of previous surgery, e.g. in a patient who has had a previous arthrodesis.
- A joint that is grossly degenerate may have limited active or passive range of movement.
- Tendon, muscle or nerve injury may preclude active movement and in these situations only passive movement can be assessed. However, be aware that the patient may use gravity or a trick movement to move the affected joint, thus misleading the examiner.
- Excessive passive joint movement or movement in abnormal planes may be the result of generalized ligamentous laxity or ligament/bony abnormality.
- Generalized ligamentous laxity can be assessed fully using Beighton's scoring system (Figure 1.4). A total score greater than or equal to 4 indicates hypermobility.

Further examination

In addition to the triad of look, feel, move, other tests specific to the part being examined may be required to enable the examiner to reach a diagnosis, e.g. the anterior draw or Lachman test for anterior cruciate ligament insufficiency. The various tests will be discussed later in this book in the respective chapters.

The examiner must be prepared to examine the joint above or below the one being examined as the patient may be presenting with referred pain. For example, a patient with a slipped upper femoral epiphysis may present with knee pain, and failure to examine the hip joint will cause the examiner to miss the diagnosis. In addition, pathology in one joint may directly affect adjacent joints.

A neurovascular assessment is also an important aspect of any examination. It is important to ascertain if there is a true neurological deficit or if neurological symptoms are mimicking musculoskeletal symptoms. In some instances (e.g. in patients with nerve palsy) it may be necessary to undertake this assessment early on in the examination after inspection.

Muscle strength is an integral part of the neurological assessment and is best carried out in a systematic manner from proximal to distal and recorded using the MRC scale (Table 1.1). It is important to understand how to differentiate between grade 2 and grade 3 by eliminating gravity (Figures 1.5 and 1.6).

Table 1.1 MRC scale for muscle strength

Grade
0 No muscle contraction
1 Flicker of contraction
2 Movement with gravity eliminated
3 Movement against gravity
4 Movement against gravity and some resistance
5 Full power

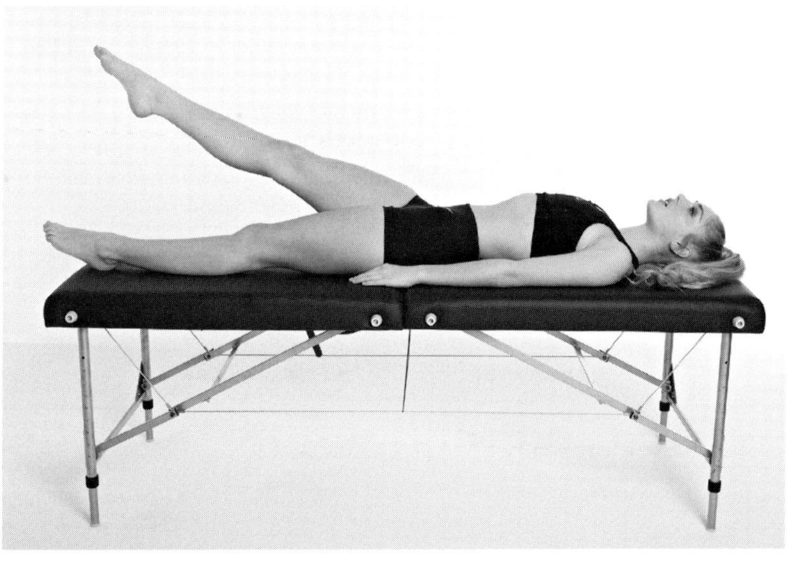

Figure 1.5 Testing MRC grade 3 muscle power of the quadriceps.

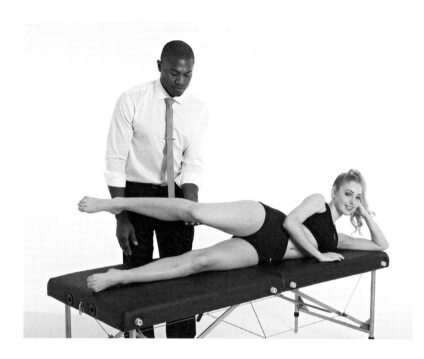

Figure 1.6 Testing MRC grade 2 power of the quadriceps with the effect of gravity eliminated.

Summary

Summary of general orthopaedic examination principles
1. Respect your patient and ensure that he or she is comfortable.
2. Give clear instructions on what you want the patient to do.
3. Fully expose the region to be examined yet maintain dignity.
4. Observe not only the region being examined but your patient as a whole.
5. Always compare both limbs.
6. When palpating a region remember to look also at the patient's face.
7. Assess both active and passive range of movement.
8. Special tests are done to help define other findings.
9. Examine the joint above and the joint below as well as performing a neurovascular assessment.
10. Do not cause pain.

Acknowledgement

We would like to acknowledge the help of Edward Oliver in the preparation of this chapter.

Further reading

Apley AG, Solomon L. *Physical Examination in Orthopaedics.* Oxford: Butterworth–Heinemann, 1997.

Beighton PH, Horan F. Orthopaedic aspects of Ehlers–Danlos syndrome. *J Bone Joint Surg* 1969;**51**:444–453.

McRae R. *Clinical Orthopaedic Examination*, 6th edition. Toronto: Churchill Livingstone, 2010.

Parvizi J. *Orthopaedic Examination Made Easy*, 1st edition. Toronto: Churchill Livingstone, 2006.

Reider B. *The Orthopaedic Physical Examination*, 2nd edition. Philadelphia: Elsevier Saunders, 2005.

Examination of the shoulder

David Limb

Introduction

There is rarely a need to carry out a comprehensive examination of the shoulder including all of the tests described in this chapter. Described below are the elements that can be used to differentiate between possible diagnoses suggested by the clinical presentation. To be successful clinically and to demonstrate competence in professional examinations, interpretation of the available history is combined with an appropriately directed examination of the shoulder. Each test answers a specific question about the state and function of the components of the shoulder or the structures that enable it to work effectively. Pieced together, the clinical examination narrows down the differential diagnosis and may direct one to supplementary investigations that prove a diagnosis. Alternatively, the clinical examination may reassure that treatment can proceed without further expensive tests, pending review to confirm the expected progress. No description of clinical examination of the shoulder can therefore be complete without mention of the history that should be elicited, as this is primarily responsible for focusing the examination to those components that move one efficiently towards the correct diagnosis.

History

Patients often present with shoulders that are painful, unstable and/or stiff. Even basic demographic details are helpful, and it is important to document these for medicolegal reasons. Age, handedness and occupation should be noted. Although an open mind should be kept at all times, instability tends to dominate in the younger age group, impingement symptoms in middle age and rotator cuff tears and arthritis in the older group.

Initially an account is gathered on how the problem began and developed and whether any treatments have been undertaken already, with a note of their outcome. The past medical history and family history may point to conditions or associations relevant to the presenting complaint, whilst the social history may be vital in formulating a treatment plan with the patient – a frail elderly patient with a moderate rotator cuff tear who is complaining of overhead weakness but no pain is very unlikely to want a cuff repair. However, the 50–year-old with the same tear and pseudoparalysis may take quite a different view.

Elements of the history are particularly useful in directing the subsequent clinical examination and these merit further attention. In particular, the surgeon should consider the history of pain, weakness, stiffness and instability.

Pain

Why do patients with shoulder problems suffer so much night pain? It is a frequent complaint, often the main presenting symptom, but elsewhere would suggest tumour or infection. Whilst tumours and infections of the shoulder do cause night pain, it is not a red flag symptom in this context as it is so common in patients with shoulder pathology.

The patient may describe pain that is accurately localized or diffuse. Neck pain radiating to the scapula or tip of the shoulder should trigger an assessment of the cervical spine, whilst radiation into the forearm and hand, particularly with parasthesiae, suggests cervical root entrapment. Pain at the tip of the scapula may suggest abdominal pathology, though posterior pain in the upper, outer part of the shoulder blade is usually glenohumeral in origin.

Examination Techniques in Orthopaedics, Second Edition, ed. Nick Harris and Fazal Ali. Published by Cambridge University Press. © Cambridge University Press 2014.

Acromioclavicular joint (ACJ) pain is classically localized to the joint itself, the patient pointing with a single finger to the source of their problem. However, it is not uncommon for ACJ pain to radiate towards the root of the neck and, furthermore, ACJ pathology may coexist with impingement syndrome, giving a wider distribution of perceived pain. The pain associated with impingement and rotator cuff disease is often diffusely felt over the deltoid region. However, the patient may report painful clicks that they localize to the anterior and lateral subacromial regions. Just as hip arthritis can present with thigh pain, shoulder arthritis commonly gives pain in the region of the deltoid insertion, at the midpoint of the humeral shaft.

There are some conditions that can be associated with excruciating pain so severe that it limits further clinical tests. Acute calcific tendonitis falls into this category, and may be confirmed by ultrasound or radiographs. The early phases of frozen shoulder can also be extremely painful and the above tests will be negative – this is particularly common in diabetic patients, and the condition also tends to be more severe and longer-lasting in this group. Also normal on radiography and ultrasound is Parsonage–Turner syndrome or brachial neuritis, with neuralgic pain that is associated with weakness and wasting in the distribution of affected peripheral nerves, unlike the nerve root distribution of cervical disc disease.

Finally, the relationship between pain and movement should be explored, not least to prevent the examiner hurting the patient subsequently. Pain that occurs only through a particular range of movement is a painful arc: rotator cuff disease, including subacromial impingement, often causes a midrange painful arc between about 60° and 120° of abduction and elevation. A high painful arc (for example, the last 30° of elevation) is typical of ACJ disorders. A painful arc with pain felt posteriorly is less common, but can occur with subscapular disorders such as enchondromata, which typically produce ratchet-like crepitus as the lesion moves over the ribs. More commonly (but less understood), abnormal muscle patterning of the scapular muscles causes tilting and the development of subscapular bursitis, causing similar subscapular crepitus. Often the patient with this problem can voluntarily exacerbate their crepitus (and pain if bursitis has developed) by tensing their shoulder girdle as they move the scapula.

Weakness

The commonest cause of perceived weakness of the shoulder is pain inhibition – if a movement hurts, the patient's brain will not let the muscles contract to produce the movement. Thus subacromial impingement may present with weakness, but this may be reversed by an injection of local anaesthetic into the subacromial space. Such diagnostic test injections are less commonly used now that diagnostic ultrasound is more freely available and can even be integrated into the clinical examination, observing deformation or bunching of the cuff as it moves under the acromion. Furthermore, weakness can be a manifestation of stiffness – if the range is not available the patient may interpret this as them not having the strength to move the arm. A history of inherited disorders or of generalized problems may alert the surgeon to rare neurological or myopathic conditions such as fascio-scapulohumeral dystrophy.

However, the majority of patients presenting to shoulder clinic (or to examinations) have a disorder either of the rotator cuff or of the nerves supplying the shoulder girdle muscles. The latter can include entrapment in the neck (cervical nerve root entrapment) or more peripherally. This includes brachial plexus injury, the assessment of which requires a detailed neurological assessment of the upper limb with mapping of all deficits to pinpoint the exact location of the lesion.

Other peripheral nerve problems that can manifest as shoulder pain and weakness include suprascapular nerve entrapment. This can occur in the suprascapular notch, in which case it is known as 'rucksack palsy' because prolonged downward traction on the shoulder has been implicated. Wasting and weakness of the supraspinatus and infraspinatus occurs and may be improved by nerve release. Interestingly, retraction of supraspinatus because of cuff tears has been suggested to cause nerve kinking in the notch, exacerbating cuff weakness with large tears. Entrapment of the suprascapular nerve can also occur as it winds round the spinoglenoid notch, often a result of pressure from cysts or ganglia related to a degenerative posterior labrum. In this case only infraspinatus is involved and the treatment relies on dealing with the cyst causing compression. Axillary nerve weakness, with deltoid wasting, may follow axillary nerve injury. Both this, and musculocutaneous nerve injury, may follow anterior shoulder dislocation.

Common things being common, however, the most frequent cause of weakness in the shoulder clinic is rotator cuff disease and, in particular, rotator cuff tears.

Stiffness

Is the shoulder really stiff, or is the patient referring to pain, which limits them to moving the shoulder slowly or with assistance? If active movements are limited check passive movements, being careful not to hurt the patient. Frozen shoulder causes restriction of both active and passive movement in all planes (global restriction). Arthritic disorders can do the same, but the latter are often associated with crepitus and radiographs demonstrate the pathology, whilst radiographs are normal in cases of frozen shoulder.

Frozen shoulder has been a loosely used term and should best be reserved for the specific condition that causes inflammation, myofibroblastic transformation and contracture associated with severe pain which, for reasons that we do not understand, eventually 'thaws out', even without treatment. So-called secondary frozen shoulder refers to stiffness associated with other pathology that is associated with fibrous scarring or contracture of the glenohumeral capsule and subacromial space and is often more resistant to complete reversal. This includes stiffness after even minimally displaced fractures or rotator cuff tears. In the latter case it is important to treat the stiffness as well as the tear – sequentially if necessary – as the rehabilitation programme will be doomed to failure if the shoulder is already stiff before a repair is carried out that typically requires a period of further relative immobility afterwards.

Instability

Laxity may be found on examination of the asymptomatic shoulder. Indeed, an assessment of generalized joint laxity is important in any patient in whom instability is suspected, and can be documented using the Beighton score (Chapter 1). Instability refers to the symptomatic inability to maintain the humeral head centred in the glenoid. Its most extreme manifestation is dislocation, though patients presenting to the shoulder clinic will not usually have a dislocated shoulder (except in the case of chronic dislocation). Rather, they will complain that they can feel the shoulder slipping out of the joint and back in, with or without a past history of dislocation. Silliman and Hawkins[1] described a simple classification that broadly categorizes patients into those likely to need surgical treatment and those who may not. TUBS (traumatic, unidirectional, Bankart, surgery) and AMBRI (atraumatic, multidirectional, bilateral, rehabilitation, inferior capsular shift) are useful aide-memoires in this respect. However, this is an oversimplification and the Stanmore classification considers three axes – traumatic structural, atraumatic structural and habitual non-structural (muscle patterning) – allowing any given patient to be plotted at a point recognizing the contribution of all factors and allowing a more holistic treatment plan, and appreciating that more than one pathology can be present.[2] Thus it is important to ask about previous dislocations and their treatment (including any previous surgery), but also about the evolution of symptoms and whether the patient can voluntarily produce subluxation or dislocation.

It should be noted that instability can present as pain in provocative positions of the arm. With fatigue in sports, in particular, anterosuperior instability can manifest as typical impingement symptoms, but these are not best addressed by subacromial decompression.

Examination

Look

Inspection of the shoulder girdle should be systematic and this requires the patient to be undressed to the waist. Garments worn for modesty should leave the scapulae visible and enquiry should be made as to any concealed scars. Observing preparation for examination may be an adjunct to the history, revealing functional difficulties in arm positioning.

The general appearance of the patient may help to identify underlying disease. The shoulder is inspected from the front, back and side. Inspection of the axilla (Figure 2.1) is also required but may more conveniently be carried out during 'move'.

Inspection of the bony contours may reveal prominence of the ACJ or sternoclavicular joint (SCJ) that could be degenerative or traumatic in origin. Deformity of the clavicle is most likely to be a consequence of past trauma. Prominence of the shoulder blade could be a result of structural problems, such as malunion or osteochondroma, but is more often positional (static winging) and will be investigated further when movements are checked.

Evidence of muscle wasting is important, though can be difficult if there is a substantial layer of subcutaneous fat. However, deltoid wasting can give a 'squared-off' appearance to the shoulder. This can be a result of axillary nerve injury, but chronic shoulder pain and stiffness will also result in deltoid wasting (Figure 2.2). Ruptured long head of biceps will make the biceps appear more prominent because of a dip appearing between the muscle and deltoid (the 'Popeye' sign – Figure 2.3), whilst pectoralis major rupture will cause loss of the anterior axillary fold.

Scapula positioning is checked from behind. Hollowing of the supraspinous and infraspinous fossae suggests tears of the supraspinatus and infraspinatus, respectively (Figure 2.4). Often this gives as good an impression of the functional impact of a rotator cuff tear as does detailed ultrasound examination of the cuff tendons.

Feel

Like inspection, palpation should proceed in a systematic manner (Figure 2.5). Start at the only synovial joint between the upper limb girdle and the trunk – the SCJ – and palpate from this, along the clavicle, to the ACJ. Pathology of the joints may cause local tenderness, but when the patient continues to flinch

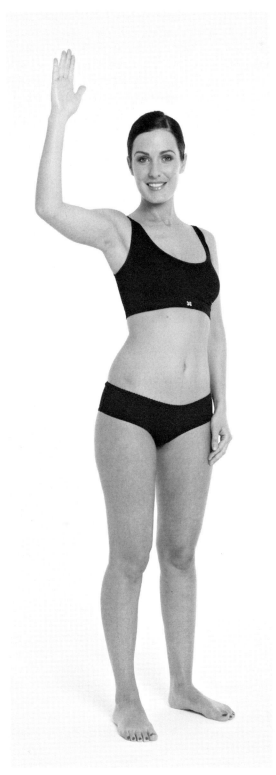

Figure 2.1 Inspect from the front, back and side. Remember to look into the axilla.

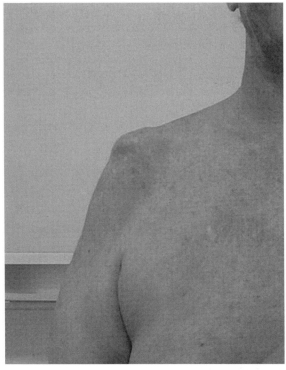

Figure 2.2 Wasting of the deltoid, in this case caused by axillary nerve injury that was the result of a previous anterior dislocation of the shoulder.

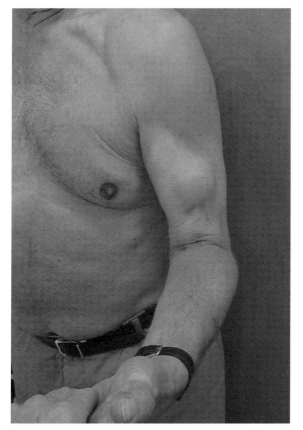

Figure 2.3 The 'Popeye' sign – prominence of the belly of the long head of biceps caused by rupture of its tendon in the intertubercular sulcus allowing distal retraction. Rupture of the distal biceps allows proximal retraction of the whole muscle belly, flattening the contour of the arm above the cubital fossa.

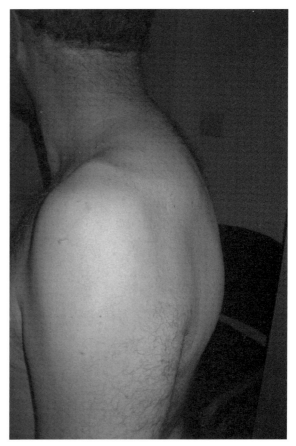

Figure 2.4 Infraspinatus and supraspinatus wasting caused by a massive rotator cuff tear.

when the clavicle, acromion and scapular spine are palpated one has to wonder on the significance of the finding and interpret tenderness with care. At the ACJ gentle ballottment by downward pressure on the distal clavicle, followed by posteriorly directed pressure on the anterior margin of the distal clavicle, can help to identify symptomatic ACJ disease (degenerative change in the ACJ is almost universal with age, so imaging is often unhelpful in identifying whether the joint is culpable as a cause of symptoms).

Tenderness along the subacromial margins can occur with impingement and cuff tears, particularly when there is bursitis, but this is a non-specific finding. Indeed, it is routine to document tenderness along the anterior and posterior joint lines and along the biceps groove about 5–7 cm distal to the tip of the acromion with the arm in neutral rotation, but diagnostic information is limited by low specificity.

Move

The 'shoulder' examination is really a composite examination of the glenohumeral (GHJ), scapulothoracic (STJ), acromioclavicular and sternoclavicular joints. It is cervical spine pathology that is most easily confused with, and commonly coexists with, shoulder girdle pathology. Hence a screening movement of the cervical spine should be performed to see if it reproduces the shoulder pain.

Movements of the shoulder are documented as the sum of movements at the GHJ, STJ, ACJ and SCJ on the position of the humerus with respect to the axis of the torso. Be careful, therefore, to eliminate any trick movements such as leaning back to increase apparent elevation of the arm. As previously noted, active movements should be measured and then a check made to see if there is any additional passive range available. All movements are measured with a

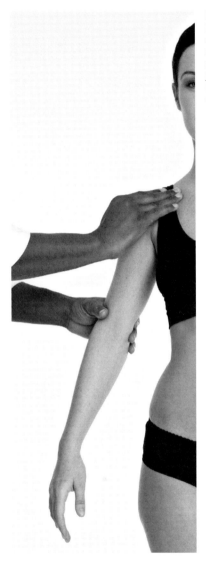

Figure 2.5
Palpate in a systematic manner starting at the sternoclavicular joint and progress laterally along the clavicle.

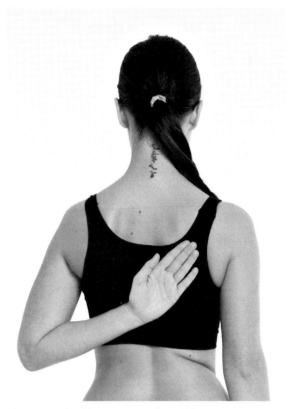

Figure 2.6 Shoulder movements: forward flexion, extension, abduction, external rotation and internal rotation as shown here.

goniometer – estimations are as poor in the shoulder as they are in any other joint and this can be a huge source of interobserver discrepancy. Note also that, although the reference planes are sagittal and coronal, this does not correspond to the plane of the GHJ because the scapula faces forwards by approximately 30°.

Shoulder flexion and extension is conventionally measured in the sagittal plane. The humerus is limited in flexion by the acromion, so if flexion of 180° **is** recorded, it is usually wrong! An angle of 160–170° is normal. Extension is often not recorded but functionally can become very important if the patient loses internal rotation – this can be compensated for by a combination of extension and adduction, another movement that is often not recorded as part of the routine shoulder examination.

Whilst adduction is not usually measured (as it can only be measured in positions of flexion and extension), abduction is recorded and any painful arc is documented. Scapular rotation coupled with external rotation of the proximal humerus (to take the greater tuberosity out of the subacromial space) allows a full 180° of this movement in normal subjects.

External rotation is measured with the arms by the side and the elbows in 90° of flexion. The neutral position is with the forearms pointing directly forwards in the sagittal plane. The 'normal' range of external rotation is very variable so should be carefully measured and recorded if any changes over time or with treatment are to be detected. Furthermore, any side-to-side difference may be significant.

Internal rotation cannot be measured in this position because the forearms become blocked by the abdomen long before the limit of internal rotation is reached. The range of internal rotation, and external rotation, can be documented with the shoulder at 90° of abduction, but note that the available range is different in this position when compared to the arms-by-the-side position. The anterosuperior capsule and rotator interval structures are under less tension at the starting position and the range of external rotation is greater, whilst the inferior glenohumeral ligaments are already lengthened in the starting position and the range of internal rotation is less. It is therefore vital to document not only the range of internal and external rotation, but the position of the shoulder when the measurements were made. To skirt around this, internal rotation is more conventionally measured in a more functional way, documenting how far behind one can reach with the tip of the thumb (greater trochanter, buttock, sacroiliac joint, L5, 4, 3, etc.) (Figure 2.6).

When measuring abduction, stand behind the patient and observe the scapulae. Scapular rhythm refers to the relative contributions of scapulothoracic and glenohumeral movement to the total range and is normally 1:2, delivered smoothly and simultaneously, with a slight predominance of glenohumeral movement in the lower range. An abnormal rhythm can arise with shoulder pathology. For example, an osteoarthritic glenohumeral joint may demonstrate little movement at the GHJ but full movement at the STJ. The contributions can be formally examined by stabilizing the scapula by manually fixing the tip of the scapula and the acromion (Figure 2.7). This will restrict abduction in the normal shoulder to about 80° with the arm in neutral rotation, or 120° if external rotation of the arm is allowed, bringing the greater tuberosity out from beneath the acromion.

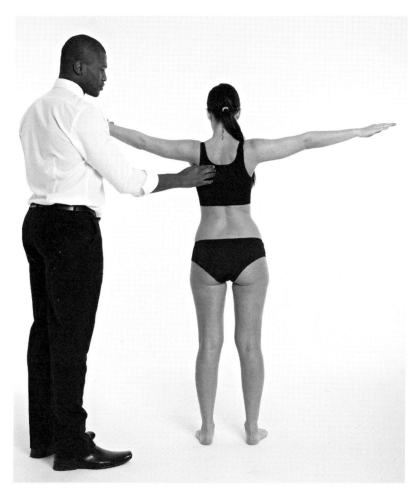

Figure 2.7 Stabilizing the scapula to separate the glenohumeral and scapulothoracic components of abduction.

Observing the rhythm of scapular movement is combined with observation for winging of the scapula. With paralysis of serratus anterior there may be gross and obvious prominence of the medial border of the scapula, but many painful conditions (such as impingement syndrome) will cause pain inhibition of groups of muscles, resulting in dynamic winging that can be quite subtle, perhaps only occurring for part of the range of movement.

Muscle testing

Rotator cuff

The muscles of the rotator cuff are tested in sequence. This may be followed by testing the deltoid and other muscles around the shoulder girdle if indicated.

Infraspinatus

Infraspinatus is the most powerful external rotator of the shoulder when the arms are by the side. In this position the patients elbows are flexed 90° and the power of external rotation is assessed (Figure 2.8). If the infraspinatus tendon is involved in a rotator cuff tear this movement is very weak. With complete weakness the patient cannot externally rotate the arm to reach up to their mouth so they compensate by abducting the shoulder and flexing the elbow to reach the mouth – the position used to sound a hunting horn (Hornblower's sign) (Figure 2.9).

Infraspinatus and teres minor, the other external rotator, can also be tested by a series of 'drop' and 'lag' tests. Bigliani et al. described a 'drop sign' in which the arm is passively, maximally externally rotated and then released. If there is severe external rotator weakness, the arm will fall into internal rotation.[3] Hertel et al.[4] described a modification of this sign in which the patient is seated with the examiner standing behind; the arm is supported at the elbow, which is held at 90°, and the shoulder is elevated 20° in the scapula plane. The shoulder is then passively placed in almost full external rotation by the examiner. The patient is asked to maintain this position actively, then the examiner releases the patient's hand. The sign is positive (an external rotation lag sign) when the forearm drops back towards neutral rotation of the shoulder. They also described a drop sign that differs from that described by Bigliani et al. in which

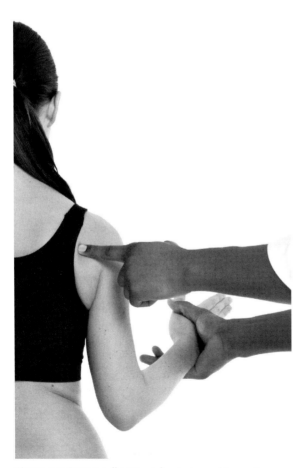

Figure 2.8 Rotator cuff: testing infraspinatus and teres minor muscles by resisting external rotation.

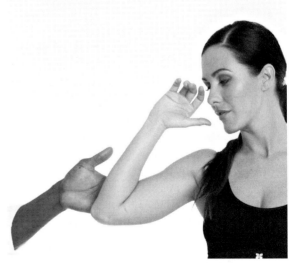

Figure 2.9 Hornblower's sign. With infraspinatus weakness the patient compensates by abducting shoulder and flexing elbow.

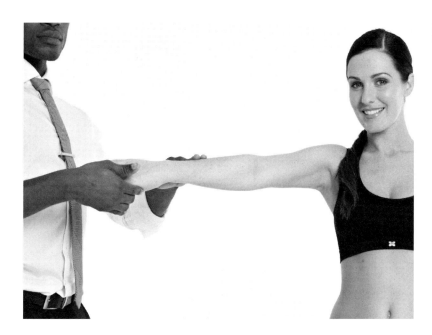

Figure 2.10 Rotator cuff: testing supraspinatus.

the arm is supported at the elbow with the shoulder elevated 90° in the scapular plane and almost fully externally rotated. Again, the patient is asked to maintain this position when the examiner releases the wrist. The sign is positive if a lag or 'drop' occurs.

Supraspinatus

Supraspinatus is an abductor of the shoulder and, despite what is taught in undergraduate anatomy, most patients with a torn supraspinatus can still initiate abduction. Furthermore, the power of abduction can be good because deltoid is also a powerful abductor. To test supraspinatus the shoulder is elevated in the plane of the scapula, 30° forwards from the coronal plane and in line with the supraspinatus muscle (Figure 2.10). A position of about 60° of abduction places the fibres of an intact supraspinatus at their ideal length for tension generation. If the arm is fully internally rotated and kept in this position the contribution of deltoid is minimized (as, if it did contract, it would cause external rotation back to the neutral position), therefore abduction of the internally rotated arm tests supraspinatus. There are several variations on this theme, all with slightly different positions, but the principle is the same. In the 'empty can test' described by Jobe and Moynes, for example, the testing conditions are as above but with 90° of abduction.[5] Kelly et al. 's modification,[6] the 'full can test' uses the same position as described by Jobe and

Moynes but uses a position of 45° external rotation rather than full internal rotation, which is less painful but has equal diagnostic accuracy.[7]

Subscapularis

Although subscapularis has the opposite action to infraspinatus, being a powerful internal rotator of the humerus when the arm is by the side, this cannot be used for testing because pectoralis major is equally strong in this respect. There are two strategies to get around this. If the patient has sufficient range then the hand is placed behind the back and from this position the strength of further internal rotation – pushing the examiner's hand away from the small of the back – is tested (Figure 2.11). This 'lift off' test[8] is the most reliable test for subscapularis but not all patients with painful shoulders can reach behind their backs. The patient is asked to keep the elbow forwards but to press their hand into their abdomen. If pectoralis major is recruited this pulls the humerus and brings the elbow back, therefore to keep the elbow forwards requires that only subscapularis is used for this internal rotation movement (Napoleon test or belly press test) (Figure 2.12).

A lag sign has also been described for the detection of subscapularis tears.[4] The hand is drawn away from the small of the back by the examiner and the patient is asked to hold their hand away from the back when it is released. The lag sign is positive if the

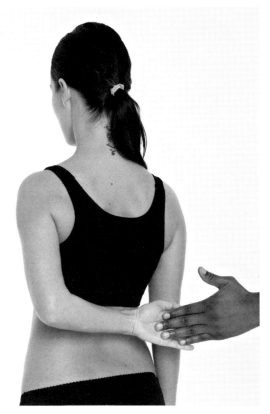

Figure 2.11 Rotator cuff: testing subscapularis.

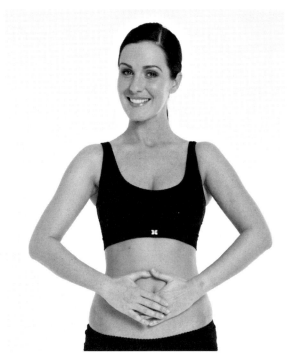

Figure 2.12 Napoleon test or belly press test for subscapularis.

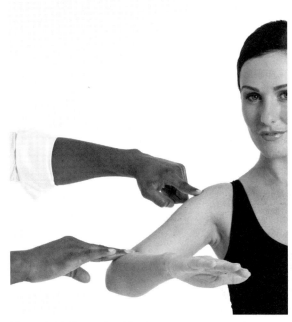

Figure 2.13 Testing the deltoid.

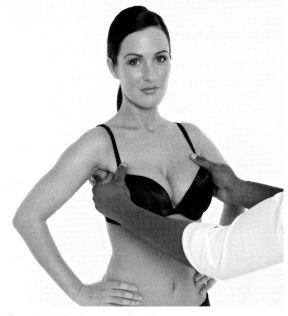

Figure 2.14 Testing pectoralis major.

patient cannot maintain the hand in this position and it falls back onto the lumbar region, suggesting subscapularis rupture.

Testing other muscles around the shoulder girdle

Test for deltoid: deltoid can be tested either with the arm by the side or, if the patient allows, in 90° of abduction, which makes visualization and palpation easier. From either of these positions, abduction, flexion and extension against resistance will lead to visible and palpable contraction of the lateral, anterior and posterior heads of deltoid, respectively (Figure 2.13).

Test for pectoralis major: hands on waist and squeeze inwards. Palpate the muscle (Figure 2.14).

Test for latissimus dorsi: downwards/backwards pressure of arm against resistance, as though climbing a ladder. Palpate muscle (Figure 2.15).

Figure 2.15 Testing latissimus dorsi.

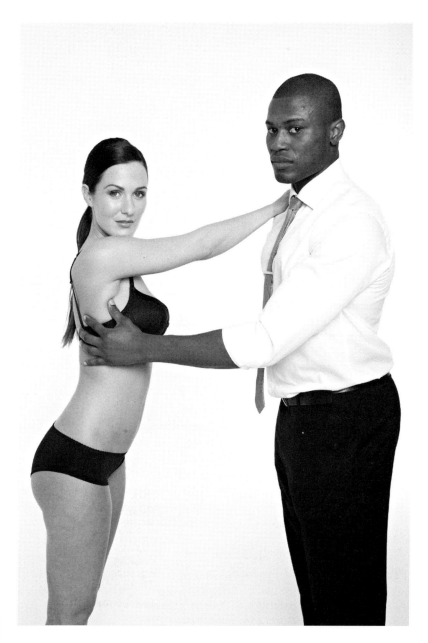

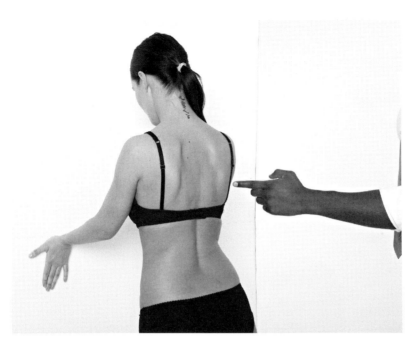

Figure 2.16 Testing serratus anterior.

Test for rhomboids: hands on hips pushing elbows back against resistance. Feel muscle.

Test for serratus anterior: patient pushes against wall with outstretched arm, the fingers and palm pointing downwards on the wall (Figure 2.16). Scapular winging is observed.

Test for trapezius: patient shrugs shoulders against resistance (Figure 2.17).

Impingement signs and tests

Neer and Welsh described an impingement sign and an impingement test. The sign[9] is elicited by passively elevating the internally rotated arm in the scapular plane whilst stabilizing the scapula (Figure 2.18). The sign is positive if pain is felt, usually in the arc of 70–120°, exacerbated by downward pressure on the scapula if necessary. Neer's test involves the subsequent instillation of local anaesthetic into the subacromial space, after which the manoeuvre is repeated. The test is positive if the impingement sign is abolished.

Hawkins and Kennedy[10] described a similar test in which the arm is elevated to the horizontal and adducted by about 10°. From this position internal rotation of the arm provokes pain in impingement syndromes (Figure 2.19). Likewise, this can be

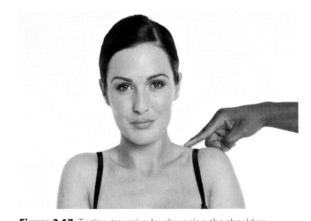

Figure 2.17 Testing trapezius by shrugging the shoulders.

repeated after subacromial infiltration of local anaesthetic, demonstrating relief of the provocation of pain.

It should be recalled that impingement is not a diagnosis in itself and the cause should be sought. For instance, in the younger patient, impingement may be caused by subtle instability of the shoulder.

Acromioclavicular joint

ACJ pathology may have been suggested by the localization of symptoms, joint tenderness and a high painful arc. Pain is provoked by elevating the arm

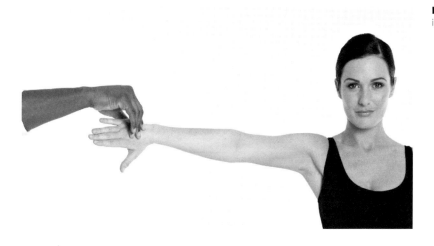

Figure 2.18 Neer's sign for impingement.

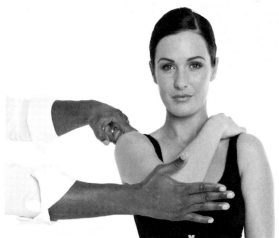

Figure 2.20 Scarf test for acromioclavicular joint pathology.

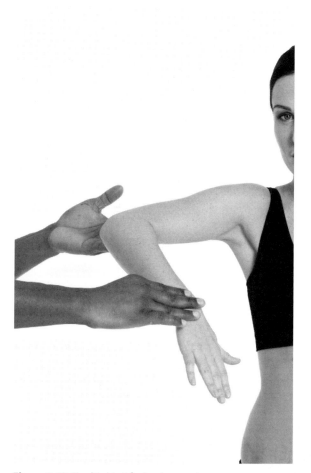

Figure 2.19 Hawkins' test for impingement.

to shoulder height then adducting across the chest (Scarf test) (Figure 2.20). In O'Brien's test[11] the arm is elevated to the horizontal, adducted by 15° and fully internally rotated. The patient is then asked to resist downward pressure exerted on the wrist (Figure 2.21). Pain felt at the ACJ in this position of testing is said to arise from the joint, though this is not a very specific test. Indeed, it has been shown to be a more sensitive test for identifying rotator cuff tears or SLAP lesions (superior labrum, anterior to posterior). To continue the theme of diagnostic test injections, this too can be repeated 5–10 minutes

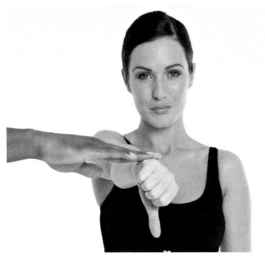

Figure 2.21 O'Brien's test can be used to detect SLAP lesions.

after injecting local anaesthetic into the ACJ. With the ready availability of ultrasound and diminishing time for assessment of patients in clinic, these test injections are less frequently carried out but remain useful. However, they should be avoided if ultrasound is to be carried out within the next day or two, as the injection fluid itself can be misinterpreted to be a bursal or joint effusion.

Biceps tendon pathology

The role of the long head of the biceps tendon is not fully understood, but inflammation of the tendon, structural damage to its insertion on the supraglenoid tubercle (SLAP tears) and structural injury to the biceps pulley, which supports the tendon as it turns from the intertubercular sulcus into the GHJ, have all been implicated as sources of pain. Several tests are available to detect biceps pathology, though all can be falsely positive in the presence of rotator cuff disease.

A rupture of the long head of biceps may have been identified by the 'Popeye sign' on inspection. In Speed's test[12] the elbow is fully extended and the forearm supinated. Anterior shoulder pain on flexion against resistance is indicative of biceps tendon pathology (Figure 2.22). Yergasson's test[11] is performed by taking the patient's hand as if to perform a handshake. With the patient's elbow by their side, held at 90° flexion, the patient is asked to attempt to twist the examiner's hand by pronation and supination of

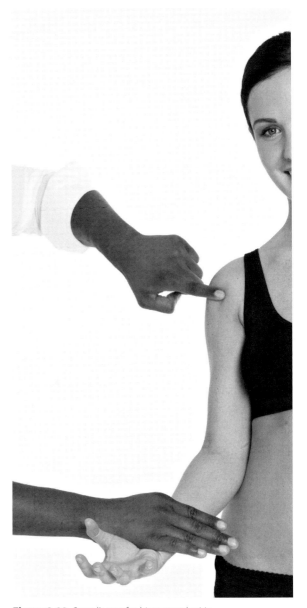

Figure 2.22 Speed's test for biceps tendonitis.

their own forearm and this is resisted. Pain provoked by resisted supination of the patient's forearm but not pronation is indicative of biceps tendon pathology. In the Crank test the shoulder is abducted to 90° and the elbow flexed to 90°. The patient is then asked to attempt to flex the elbow further against resistance, again provoking pain with biceps tendon pathology.

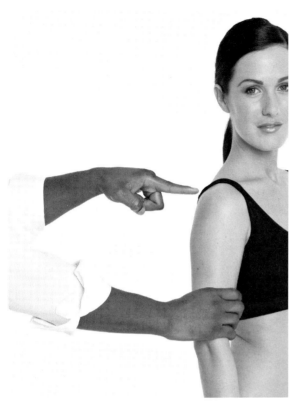

Figure 2.23 Testing for the sulcus sign.

Instability testing

Instability may be suggested by the history. However, even in cases of recurrent anterior dislocation, a systematic examination for evidence of instability in each direction is required as there can be overlap of traumatic and atraumatic causes and coexistence of constitutional and traumatic contributory factors. It is useful in all cases to compare findings with the opposite shoulder. Evidence of generalized joint laxity may also be sought, expressed by the Beighton score. Anterior and posterior instability should be sought and either, or both, in combination with inferior laxity is termed multidirectional instability.

Inferior laxity can be identified by the presence of a sulcus sign, elicited by passive downward traction on the humerus in neutral rotation (Figures 2.23 and 2.24). If this is also present in external rotation it implies incompetence of the rotator interval structures (coracohumeral ligament and superior glenohumeral ligament).

The anterior and posterior capsulolabral structures can be tested in a similar manner using load

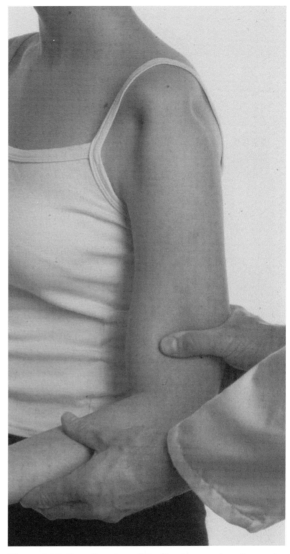

Figure 2.24 The sulcus sign, elicited by downward traction on the humerus causing inferior subluxation of the humeral head.

and shift tests (Figure 2.25). The examiner stands behind the patient and stabilizes the scapula by applying the thumb to the posterior acromion and the index finger on the coracoid process, using the examiner's left hand for testing the right shoulder and vice versa. The proximal humerus is grasped close to the humeral head between the thumb posteriorly and the index and middle fingers anteriorly. The humeral head is then translated backwards and forwards and the amount of passive movement between the humeral head and glenoid is estimated. The humeral head can be felt to glide up to the

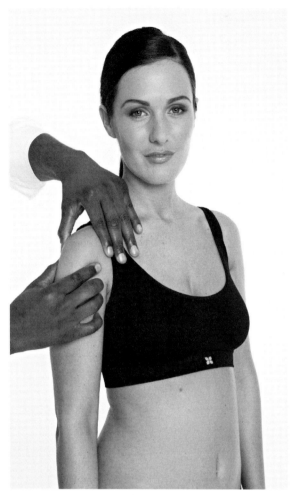

Figure 2.25 The load and shift test for anterior–posterior instability.

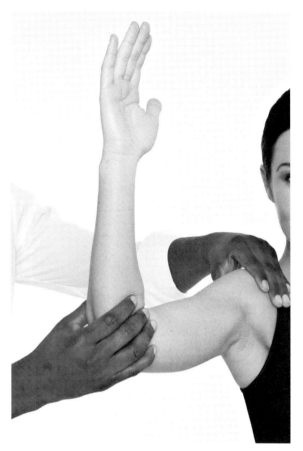

Figure 2.26 The anterior apprehension test.

glenoid rim, moving laterally as it does, perch and then, with extreme laxity, pass beyond and begin to medialize again. The extent to which it translates is used to categorize the laxity. Pain or clicks during this test can be indicative of labral tears or damage to the glenoid rim.

Further evidence of anterior and posterior instability can be gained with the apprehension tests (though the posterior test may not be associated with much in the way of apprehension).

The anterior apprehension test can be performed with the patient seated or lying down, with the shoulder to be tested at the edge of the couch (Figure 2.26). The shoulder is abducted to 90° and the elbow flexed to 90°. Gentle passive external rotation from

this position, with or without gentle anterior pressure applied to the back of the humeral head, can make the patient fearful that dislocation will occur if the apprehension test is positive. Indeed, they have good reason – this test can provoke dislocation if carried out too forcefully or in the presence of an engaging Hill–Sachs lesion. To refine this test further in the seated position, gentle anterior pressure on the back of the humeral head can be maintained whilst external rotation is carried out to the point at which involuntary contraction of pectoralis major occurs or the patient stops the examination due to apprehension. This can be repeated at various positions of abduction, for example 60, 90 and 120°, to give more information on the likely extent of labral detachment (the more inferiorly the detachment extends, the greater degree of abduction into which

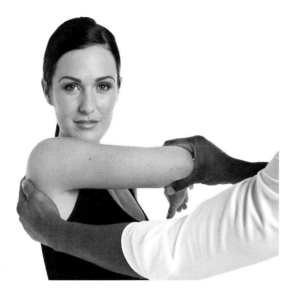

Figure 2.27 The posterior apprehension test.

apprehension persists or the more extensive is the Hill–Sachs lesion).

The posterior apprehension test puts the arm into a position that provokes posterior subluxation or dislocation – achieved by horizontal adduction of the internally rotated arm whilst axial load is applied along the humerus (Figure 2.27). Even if apprehension does not occur or is equivocal, axial load should be maintained as the arm is brought out of internal rotation and adduction. Relocation of the subluxed humeral head may be felt, analogous to the Barlow/Ortolani combination in testing infant hips.

Conclusion

Clinical examination of the shoulder adds to diagnostic information gathered when taking a history and directs one to appropriate further investigations or treatments. However, the signs have to be interpreted in context, as none of the tests described above has perfect sensitivity or specificity. None are truly diagnostic and a meta-analysis suggested that no test for impingement or ACJ pathology demonstrated sufficient diagnostic accuracy[12]. A holistic view should be taken when examining a patient after listening to their description of the problems they are experiencing with their shoulder.

Summary

Summary of shoulder examination
Step 1 Stand the patient
Step 2 Look
Step 3 Feel
Step 4 Move
Step 5 Examine muscles • Rotator cuff • Consider other muscles (e.g. deltoid, pectoralis major, latissimus dorsi, rhomboids, trapezius and serratus anterior)
Step 6 Impingement tests
Step 7 Sit patient (or lie) and perform: Instability tests

Stand and look

Stand the patient and look from the front. Ask him or her to do a quick screen of neck movements and ask whether this reproduces the shoulder pain. Look laterally. Look in to the axilla and look behind, describing any wasting, scars, etc.

Feel

Feel the bony prominences, starting from the SCJ and across the clavicle. Feel the coracoid and feel the biceps tendon and the scapular spine.

Move

Ask the patient to move. Forward flexion, abduction, internal rotation and external rotation are all done by demonstrating this to the patient. Abduction must be done looking from the front and from behind, observing scapular thoracic movement.

Test muscles

When testing the muscles test them as a separate entity, i.e. test the four muscles of the rotator cuff together, then test the muscles of the shoulder girdle separately. Also, do not combine muscle testing with other tests such as Neer's sign.

First the muscles of the rotator cuff are tested. **Four** muscles:

- Supraspinatus using Jobe's test.
- Infraspinatus and teres minor together by assessing external rotation. Teres minor weakness isolated by looking for Hornblower's sign.
- Subscapularis by performing the Gerber's lift off test.

At this point consider assessing other muscles of the shoulder girdle. It is not necessary in all cases to assess these muscles, but in some instances, especially if there is muscle wasting or weakness, it may be wise to do so:

- from the front of the patient assess deltoids, pectoralis major and latissimus dorsi;
- from the back assess trapezius, rhomboids and serratus anterior.

Impingement

- Neer's sign and/or Hawkins' test for subacromial impingement.
- Scarf test for ACJ pathology
- Speed's or Yergasson's test for biceps tendonitis.
- O'Brien's test for SLAP lesions.

Instability

For this it is wise to lie the patient down (if there is no couch then sit the patient and make him or her comfortable) and to ask whether there is instability of the shoulder.

Tests performed commonly for instability are:

- sulcus sign;
- anterior and posterior draw test (load and shift);
- anterior apprehension;
- posterior apprehension.

Note: if the patient has signs of multidirectional instability then test for generalized laxity (Beighton's test).

References

1 Silliman JF, Hawkins RJ. Classification and physical diagnosis of instability of the shoulder. *Clin Orth* 1993; **291**:7–19.

2 Lewis A, Kitamura T, Bayley JIL. The classification of shoulder instability: new light through old windows! *Current Orthopaedics* 2004;**18**(2):97–108.

3 Bigliani LU, Cordasco FA, McIlveen SJ, Musso ES. Operative treatment of massive rotator cuff tears: long term results. *J Shoulder Elbow Surg* 1992;**1**:120–130.

4 Hertel R, Ballmer FT, Lambert SM, Gerber C. Lag signs in the diagnosis of rotator cuff rupture.

J Shoulder Elbow Surg 1996;**5**(4): 307–313

5 Jobe FW, Moynes DR. Delineation of diagnostic criteria and a rehabilitation program for rotator cuff injuries. *Am J Sports Med* 1982;**10**:336–339.

6 Kelly BT, Kadrmas WR, Speer KP. The manual muscle examination for rotator cuff strength: an electromyographic investigation. *Am J Sports Med* 1996;**24**: 581–588.

7 Itoi E, Kido T, Sano A, Masakazu U, Sato K. Which is the more useful, the "full can test" or the "empty can test", in detecting the torn supraspinatus tendon? *Am J Sports Med* 1999;**27**(**1**): 65–68.

8 Gerber C, Krushell RJ. Isolated tears of the subscapularis muscle: clinical features in sixteen cases. *J Bone Joint Surg (Br)* 1991; **73B**:389–399.

9 Neer CS II, Welsh PR. The shoulder in sports. *Orthop Clin North Am* 1977;**8**:583–591.

10 Hawkins RJ, Kennedy JC. Impingement syndromes in athletes. *Am J Sports Med* 1980;**8**:151–157.

11 Yergasson RM. Supination sign. *J Bone Joint Surg (Br)* 1931;**13**:160.

12 Hegedus EJ, Goode A, Campbell S, *et al.* Physical examination tests of the shoulder: a systematic review with meta-analysis of individual tests. *Br J Sports Med* 2008;**42**:80–92.

Chapter 3

Examination of the elbow

Amjid Ali and David Stanley

As with the examination of all other joints in the body, a carefully taken and detailed clinical history will often lead the clinician to a provisional diagnosis of the cause of the patient's elbow problem.

It is important that, as the patient describes the symptoms, the clinician interprets the information in the light of the local anatomy, most of which, because the elbow is a superficial joint, can be palpated and assessed during the examination.

History

It is always essential when taking a history to record the patient's age, sex and hand dominance.

Age will give an immediate clue as to the likelihood of certain conditions being responsible for the patient's complaints. For example, osteochondritis dissecans may be the underlying cause of elbow locking in a young patient, whereas the same symptom in an older patient is more likely to be caused by loose body formation associated with degenerative disease.

The elbow may be the first presenting site of rheumatoid arthritis and, since this occurs more commonly in women, the sex of the patient should alert one to the possibility of this diagnosis if the initial symptoms are pain and slight swelling.

Hand dominance is of importance since a disorder of the dominant elbow may result in the patient's inability to work, participate in sporting activity or undertake activities of daily living.

In addition to the current symptoms it is important to enquire about the patient's previous medical health, particularly with regard to whether there is any history of previous similar problems. Enquiry should also be made with regard to previous trauma, occupation and current sporting activity.[1]

Presenting symptoms

Most patients with elbow disorders present with pain, often associated with tenderness, or reduced elbow movement. In addition, intermittent swelling and locking may also occur. More unusually, recurrent instability of the elbow is a significant problem. Combinations of these symptoms are not infrequent.

The nature of the patient's pain, together with its location and frequency, should be noted. It is important to record whether the pain is associated with movement and whether or not there is a history of pain radiation. For example, patients with ulnar nerve entrapment may experience local pain and tenderness at the elbow together with pain radiation down into the hand affecting the little and ring fingers, often with intermittent pins and needles or numbness.

Reduced elbow movement can be the result of a variety of conditions but is perhaps more commonly seen after elbow trauma or as a result of degenerative and inflammatory arthropathies. Loose bodies within the elbow joint may be another cause of reduced elbow movement and this pathology is also often associated with intermittent elbow locking.

Although rare, recurrent instability of the elbow does occur following elbow trauma, particularly if the coronoid process has been damaged or the collateral ligaments torn. Instability may also be a feature of inflammatory arthropathy, especially when the disease has resulted in significant bony destruction.

Symptoms of crepitus are not often reported by the patient and should be specifically asked about since this may indicate mechanical derangement of the elbow or an inflammatory arthropathy.

Examination Techniques in Orthopaedics, Second Edition, ed. Nick Harris and Fazal Ali. Published by Cambridge University Press. © Cambridge University Press 2014.

As with all upper limb disorders it is essential to ask the patient specifically about neck symptoms since, at times, cervical spine pathology may result in symptoms referable to the elbow.

General health

It is of relevance to enquire about the patient's general health since this may indicate a generalized musculo-skeletal disorder. In addition, enquiry as to the patient's family history may reveal problems such as haemophilia or osteochondromatosis.

The patient's occupation is of relevance since there is some evidence to suggest that heavy manual work may be associated with degenerative change within the elbow joint.[2] Similarly, an enquiry with regard to sporting activity is of importance. Throwing athletes may develop symptoms of ulnar collateral ligament insufficiency, occurring primarily during the late cocking and early acceleration phases of the throwing movement. Other athletes who undertake recurrent flexion and extension movements of the elbow, i.e. boxers, may develop posterior elbow impingement resulting from recurrent impact of the tip of the olecranon into the olecranon fossa.

Examination

Inspection

It is important to note the posture in which the patient holds the elbow. A painful elbow will often be protected with the arm being held adjacent to the patient's body, whilst patients who are unable to extend the elbow fully often find it most comfortable resting the arm by placing the hand in a trouser pocket.

Inspection should also include a close assessment of the elbow for evidence of previous scars, either traumatic or surgical, or the presence of elbow swelling such as will occur with an acute injury, inflammatory arthritis or a neoplastic lesion (Figure 3.1). Rheumatoid nodules may be noted on the extensor aspect of the elbow. Always remember to inspect the medial aspect of the elbow.

The elbow carrying angle should be assessed with the elbow in full extension. If this is not possible because of elbow pathology then the assessment of the carrying angle is compromised.

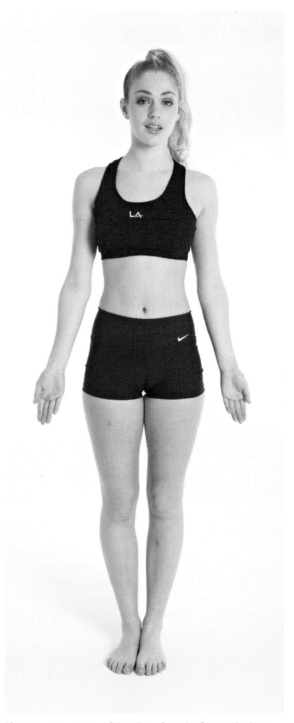

Figure 3.1 Inspection of the elbow from the front and side is followed by inspection from behind and medially. From the front the carrying angle is noted.

(a)

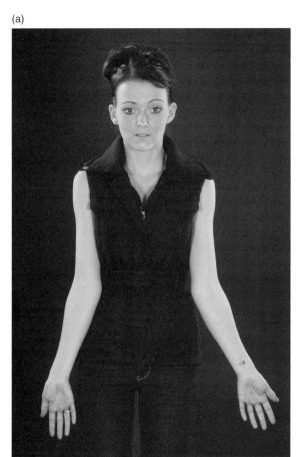

(b)

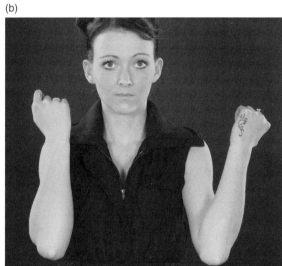

(c)

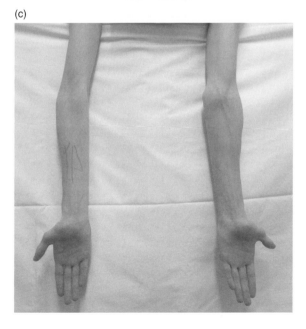

Figure 3.2 **a** Cubitus valgus from previous lateral condyle fracture of humerus. **b** Note that the valgus is maintained even with flexion of the elbow. **c** Gunstock deformity in right arm seen in a patient with a previous supracondylar fracture during childhood.

Although the carrying angle varies, the average valgus angulation is 10° in males and 15° in females. An increase in valgus angulation may result from a previous bony injury to the lateral distal humerus (Figures 3.2a, b).

Varus deformity is always abnormal and most commonly occurs as the result of a supracondylar fracture in childhood or a growth arrest on the medial side of the distal humerus (Figure 3.2c).

Movement

Movement of the elbow can only adequately be assessed in a patient whose top clothes have been removed. It is important to compare both upper limbs to identify subtle changes in elbow movement clearly.

It should be noted that when the elbow is flexed from the fully extended position the carrying angle changes from being valgus to varus.[3]

Flexion/extension

With the forearms supinated and extended the normal range of movement is from 0 to 140° of flexion (Figure 3.3). Up to 10° of hyperextension (recorded as a negative integer) is not abnormal but hyperextension beyond that level is suggestive of hypermobility or previous bony injury.

Loss of full extension is often the earliest sign of an intra-articular elbow abnormality.

A discrepancy between the passive and active range of movement is suggestive of either a musculotendinous or neurological abnormality.

Forearm rotation

Forearm rotation is assessed with both elbows flexed to 90° and with the arms adducted to the body (Figure 3.4). This prevents compensatory shoulder movement.

Variation in supination and pronation movement occurs in normal patients, although the average range of supination is 85° whilst pronation is normally a few degrees less.

Rotational deformity

Rotational deformity is often not appreciated and results from either an abnormality of the shoulder or humerus. If both shoulders are normal, an asymmetric range of rotation is indicative of a humeral rotational deformity. This may result from previous humeral fractures. The deformity is best demonstrated by the technique described by Yamamoto et al.[4]

The examiner stands behind the patient with the elbow flexed to 90° and the forearm behind the back. With the patient bent forward and the shoulder in full extension the forearm is lifted maximally, resulting in maximal internal rotation. Difference

(a)

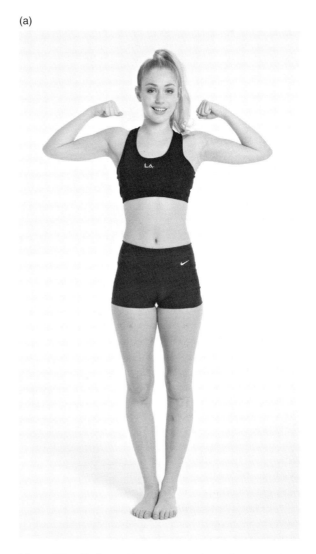

Figure 3.3 a Flexion and **b** extension can be easily compared when the arms are abducted.

(b)

Figure 3.3 (*cont.*)

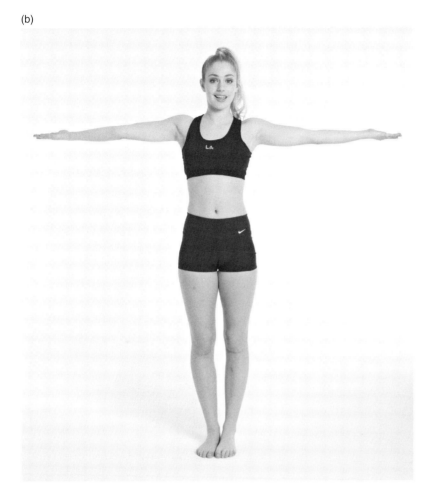

in the internal rotation angle of the two arms can be measured by the angle between the forearm and the horizontal of the back. This angle is frequently increased in malunited supracondylar fractures (Figure 3.5).

Strength

Although detailed assessment of muscle strength is not possible in the setting of the consulting room it is possible to obtain a gross assessment of muscle strength by comparing both arms.

Flexion is tested with the elbow flexed to 90° and the forearm in neutral rotation. Resistance to the flexion movement is applied and the two arms compared.

Extension is tested with the arm in a similar position but on this occasion resistance to extension movement is provided.

Pronation and supination strength is assessed with the elbows flexed to 90° and in neutral rotation. The movement under test is resisted. Normally supination is slightly stronger than pronation.

Palpation

A systematic approach to examination of the elbow must be developed. Much of the elbow is subcutaneous and therefore, by careful examination, most of the structures likely to be causing the patient's symptoms can be individually examined and assessed.

The lateral and anterior aspects of the elbow can be palpated with the examiner standing in front of the patient whilst the medial and posterior aspects of the elbow are best examined from behind with the shoulder slightly abducted and extended.

(b)

(a)

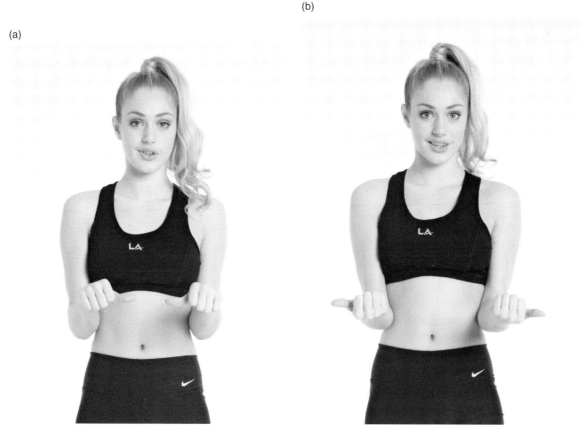

Figure 3.4 The range of **a** pronation and **b** supination is best assessed with the elbows held against the sides to minimize compensation from the shoulders.

Lateral

Examination of the lateral aspect of the elbow joint begins at the lateral supracondylar ridge (Figure 3.6). This is easily palpable. Examination should extend down the ridge to the lateral epicondyle, common extensor origin and lateral collateral ligament.

The extensor carpi radialis brevis and extensor carpi radialis longus muscles can be assessed by resisted wrist extension in neutral and radial deviation, respectively. Tenderness, particularly at the site of the extensor carpi radialis brevis, should alert the clinician to a possible diagnosis of lateral epicondylitis or tennis elbow.[5]

The capitellar joint line should be palpated since tenderness and discomfort at this site may indicate an articular injury or the presence of osteochondritis dissecans.

Inspection of the infracondylar recess between the lateral condyle and radial head will normally reveal a small sulcus. This is obliterated by fluid or synovial distension. Palpation of the area will reveal a boggy swelling if due to synovial hypertrophy while fluctuation is noted if fluid is within the joint.

The radial head is best appreciated during pronation and supination movement of the forearm. The orientation of the radial head to the capitellum should be determined and in all positions of the elbow and forearm the radial head should line up against the capitellum. Congenital or post-traumatic dislocation of the radial head (lateral, posterior or anterior) will be easily appreciated at this stage.[6]

In the presence of a recent injury palpable crepitus over the radial head together with pain on rotation movements of the forearm is usually indicative of a radial head fracture, although at times there may also be an associated capitellar injury. In the absence of a recent injury, pain and crepitus at the radiocapitellar joint is usually indicative of degenerative change. The symptoms may be exacerbated by asking the patient to grip the examiner's fingers during forearm rotation.

Anterior

Anteriorly the brachioradialis muscle, the biceps tendon together with the lacertus fibrosus, the brachial artery and the median nerve can be palpated from lateral to medial. It is therefore important to know the anatomical relationship of these structures (Figure 3.7).

Although uncommon, myositis ossificans may occur after elbow dislocation and may be palpated as an abnormal hard swelling during examination of the anterior aspect of the elbow joint.[7]

Another uncommon condition that may be appreciated on anterior elbow palpation is rupture of the insertion of the biceps tendon (Figure 3.8a).[8] The patient will normally present with a history of recent injury, most frequently caused by an eccentric load on the supinated forearm. Examination of the arm reveals a retracted biceps with the muscle bulge appearing more proximally in the arm as opposed to the more common long head of biceps rupture where the muscle bulge is distal. Assessment of power usually reveals moderate loss of flexion strength at the elbow but more marked weakness of supination. The 'hook' test will demonstrate the presence or absence of the distal biceps tendon at the anterior aspect of the elbow (Figure 3.8b).

Medial

Tenderness on palpation of the medial epicondyle and origin of the common flexors will indicate medial epicondylitis, whilst tenderness over the belly of pronator teres should suggest the diagnosis of pronator syndrome.[9] Clinical features of this syndrome are often rather vague. They consist primarily of diffuse proximal forearm discomfort and weakness which, in addition, may be associated with distal sensory changes in the distribution of the median nerve. Phalen's test and Tinel's sign are negative at the wrist whilst percussion over the median nerve at the elbow results in tingling distally.

Provocation tests, when positive, are helpful in confirming the diagnosis. These include resisted pronation for 60 seconds, resisted elbow flexion and forearm supination and resisted middle finger flexion at the proximal interphalangeal joint.

The ulnar nerve should be palpated and can be easily felt behind the medial epicondyle (Figure 3.9a). It should be remembered that in up to 10% of patients the ulnar nerve may sublux anteriorly and it is important to identify the position of the ulnar nerve during flexion and extension movements of the elbow (Figure 3.9b). A subluxing ulnar nerve may give rise to medial elbow pain.

(a)

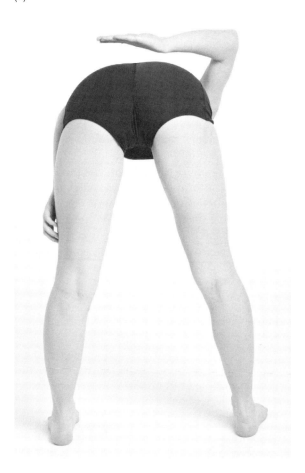

Figure 3.5 a and **b** The assessment of rotational deformity. The patient is bent forward. The shoulder is fully extended and the elbow flexed to 90°. If there is no rotational deformity the forearm is parallel to the ground. If there is increased internal rotation in the humerus then the acute angle between the line of the forearm and the horizontal gives a measure of the internal rotation deformity.

(b)

Figure 3.5 (*cont.*)

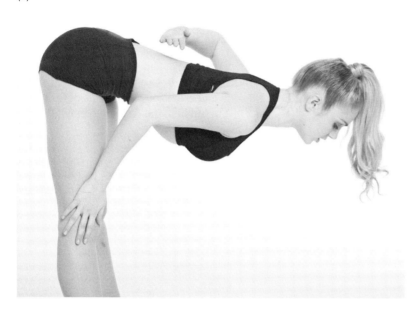

More commonly, compression of the ulnar nerve gives rise to sensory and/or motor symptoms.[10] These may occur secondary to degenerative or inflammatory arthritis, medial epicondylitis, elbow instability and fracture dislocations. The nerve is most commonly compressed at the cubital tunnel and between the two heads of flexor carpi ulnaris. Tinel's sign is usually positive at the point of maximal nerve tenderness.

Posterior

With the elbow extended the tip of the olecranon process and the medial and lateral epicondyles form a straight line. On flexion of the elbow to 90° these landmarks form an isosceles triangle (Figure 3.10). Any abnormality of this normal arrangement is suggestive of previous bony injury.

With the arm extended the triceps insertion onto the olecranon can be palpated and the integrity of the triceps tested by resisted extension. Tenderness on this manoeuvre may represent a partial tear of the triceps whilst an inability to extend against gravity is indicative of a complete triceps avulsion.[11]

The olecranon fossa can be palpated with the elbow flexed to 30°. In the thin patient it is occasionally possible to palpate a loose body within the fossa.

Examination of the olecranon bursa may reveal a bursitis or indicate the presence of rheumatoid nodules.

Provocation tests

Lateral epicondylitis

Specific provocation tests that can be performed to help confirm the diagnosis are as follows.[12]

1. With the wrist in neutral, resisted wrist extension results in localized pain over the lateral epicondyle. Pain may also occur if the test is undertaken with the wrist in extension and radial deviation and on resisted extension of the middle finger (Figure 3.11).

2. Passive volar flexion of the wrist with elbow extension and pronation will also cause pain at the lateral epicondyle. Pinch grip, particularly between the thumb and middle finger, is often weak and painful.

Medial epicondylitis

This is characterized by tenderness of the common flexor origin at the medial epicondyle. Provocation tests include the following.

(a)

(b)

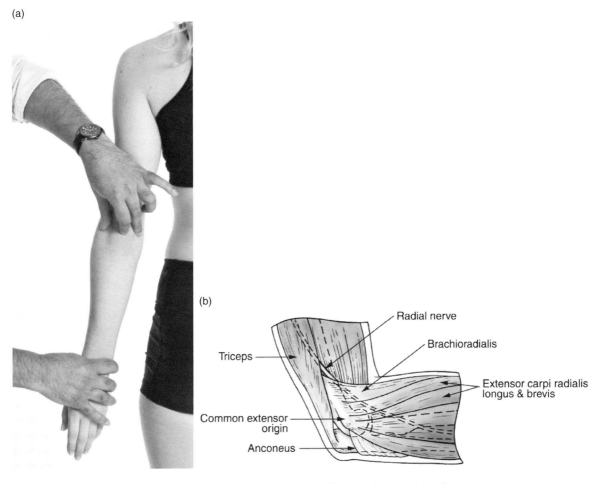

Triceps

Radial nerve

Brachioradialis

Extensor carpi radialis
longus & brevis

Common extensor
origin

Anconeus

Figure 3.6 a Palpation of the lateral aspect of the elbow. **b** The anatomy of the lateral aspect of the elbow.

1. Resisted wrist flexion causes pain at the medial epicondyle (Figure 3.12).
2. Passive extension of the wrist and elbow results in pain at the medial epicondyle.
3. Clenching of the fist may also cause pain at the medial epicondyle.

Impingement

Elbow impingement most commonly occurs in the posterior compartment of the elbow joint but can also occur anteriorly.

In the posterior compartment the symptoms are normally associated with osteophytic changes at the tip of the olecranon which impinge on the olecranon fossa during extension. Loose bodies within the olecranon fossa may produce similar symptoms in the absence of osteophytic change.

Clinically there is often a history of repetitive hyperextension movements of the elbow.

The condition can be clinically demonstrated as follows: with the patient's elbow just short of full extension, applying a gentle, rapid passive extension force reproduces the posterior pain.

Anterior impingement occurs most commonly due to osteophytes on the coronoid process impinging into the coronoid fossa. Occasionally, anterior impingement is the result of osteophytic change within the radial fossa such that on full flexion the radial head impinges with the osteophytes.

The condition can be clinically demonstrated as follows: with the patient's elbow just short of full

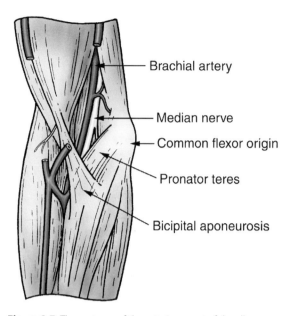

- Brachial artery
- Median nerve
- Common flexor origin
- Pronator teres
- Bicipital aponeurosis

Figure 3.7 The anatomy of the anterior aspect of the elbow.

flexion, applying a gentle, rapid passive flexion force reproduces the anterior pain.

Instability of the elbow
Varus instability

The lateral collateral ligament consists of the radial collateral ligament and the lateral ulnar collateral ligament.

To assess varus instability the elbow should be flexed to approximately 30° to unlock the olecranon from its fossa. In addition, this manoeuvre relaxes the anterior capsule. Varus stress is then applied across the elbow joint with the humerus in full internal rotation to lock the shoulder.[13] In the presence of varus instability the gap between the capitellum and radial head will increase (Figure 3.13). This can often be appreciated by clinical examination but can more easily be confirmed if the procedure is undertaken under image intensification. The elbow under examination should be compared with the normal side.

(a)

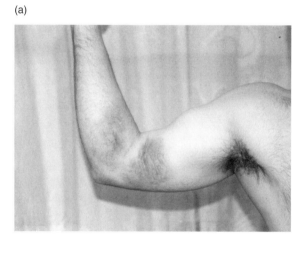

(b)

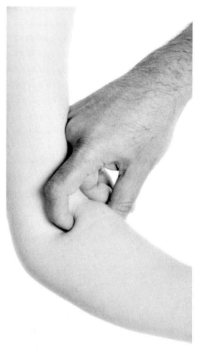

Figure 3.8 a Rupture of the insertion of the biceps. Note the proximal position of the biceps muscle. **b** Demonstration of the 'hook test'. Ask the patient to actively supinate the forearm and hook around the biceps insertion from the lateral side.

(a)

(b)

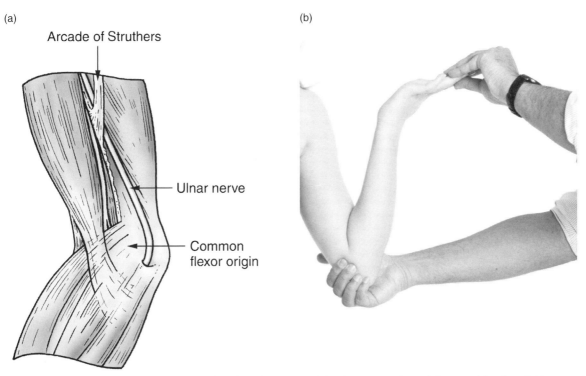

Figure 3.9 **a** The anatomy of the medial aspect of the elbow. **b** Palpation of the ulnar nerve at the medial aspect of the elbow. Subluxation of the ulnar nerve may be picked up on flexion and extension of the elbow.

(a)

(b)

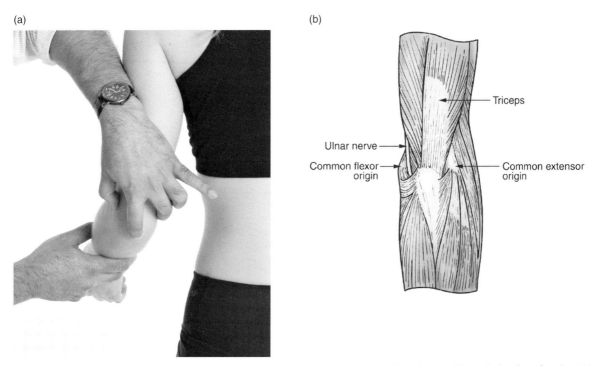

Figure 3.10 **a** The bony relationship of the tip of the olecranon process to the medial and lateral epicondyles with the elbow flexed to 90°. Here an isosceles triangle is formed. **b** The anatomy of the posterior aspect of the elbow.

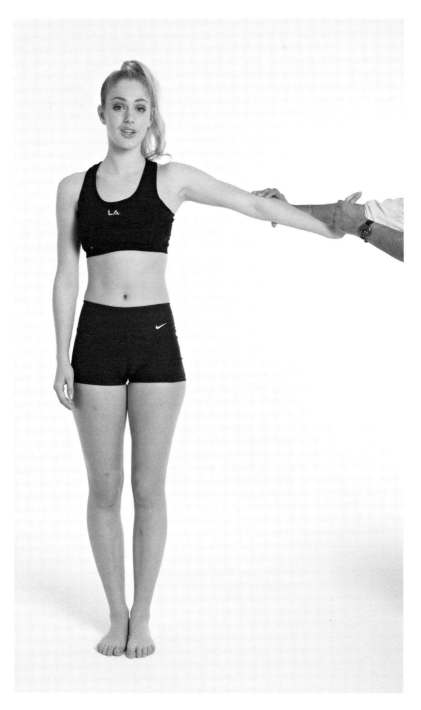

Figure 3.11 Provocation testing for lateral epicondylitis.

Valgus instability

Valgus instability is most commonly seen in throwing athletes. Assessment of the ulnar collateral ligament is best undertaken with the patient seated and the patient's forearm held securely between the examiner's arm and trunk. The patient's elbow is flexed to approximately 30° to unlock the olecranon from its fossa and then the ulnar collateral ligament is palpated whilst a valgus stress is applied to the elbow. External rotation of the humerus will lock the

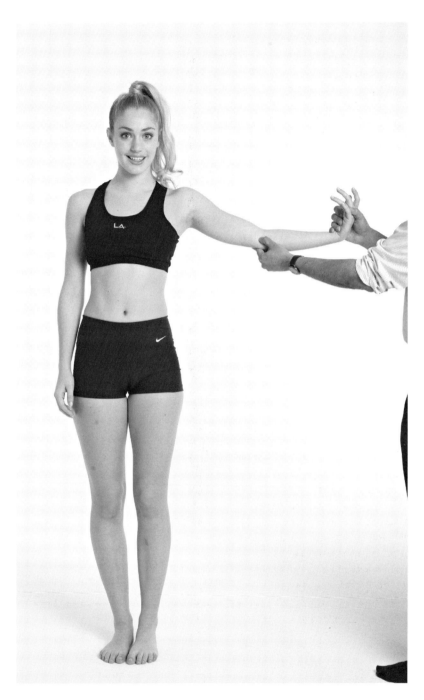

Figure 3.12 Provocation testing for medial epicondylitis.

shoulder at the same time. Opening of the elbow, local pain and tenderness are compatible with an ulnar collateral ligament injury (Figure 3.14).

Tears in continuity without gross instability can be assessed by the method described by O'Brien.[14] This involves holding the patient's thumb and fully flexing the elbow whilst a valgus stress is applied to the elbow joint.

Rotatory instability

Posterolateral rotatory instability results from insufficiency of the lateral ulnar collateral ligament (LUCL).

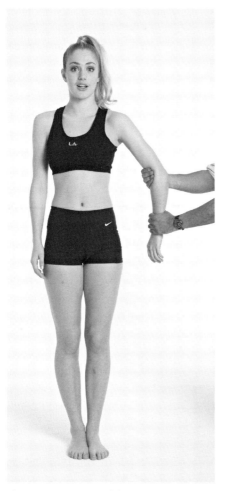

Figure 3.13 Varus instability testing. Varus stress is applied across the elbow with the humerus in full internal rotation. If instability is present the gap between the capitellum and radial head increases.

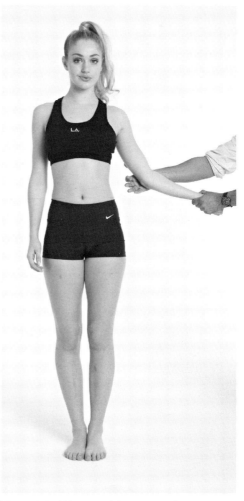

Figure 3.14 Valgus instability testing. Valgus stress is applied across the elbow with the humerus in full external rotation.

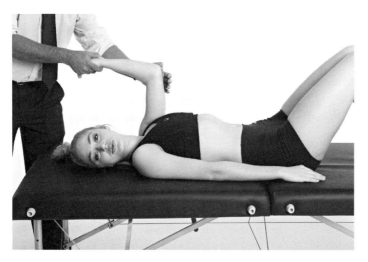

Figure 3.15 The lateral pivot shift test. With the patient lying supine and the arm above the head and forearm supinated, a valgus force with axial compression is applied to the elbow. Subluxation produces a prominence over the radial head and a dimple in the skin behind it. Further extension causes a reduction to occur with a palpable, audible, clunk.

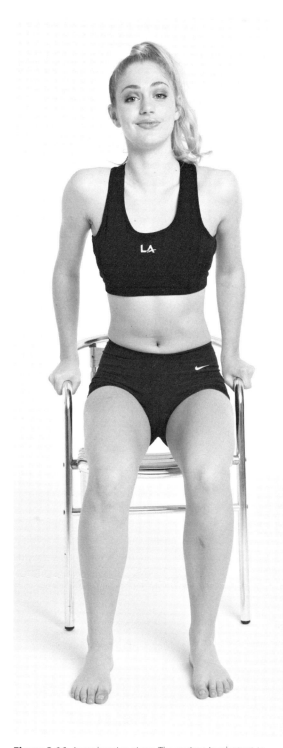

The most sensitive clinical method of assessing insufficiency of the LUCL is the lateral pivot shift test which is usually performed under general anaesthesia with image intensifier screening. The patient is positioned supine with the shoulder and elbow flexed to 90°. The patient's forearm is fully supinated and the examiner holds the patient's wrist and forearm and slowly extends the elbow whilst applying a valgus and axial compression force. Subluxation of the radius and ulna from the humerus causes a prominence posterolaterally over the radial head and a dimple between the radial head and the capitellum. When the elbow is at approximately 45° of flexion the ulna suddenly reduces with a palpable and visible clunk (Figure 3.15).[15]

Apprehension signs

Asking a patient to rise from a chair using their arms to push them into the standing position may reproduce symptoms of instability. In such a situation the patient is reluctant to extend the elbow fully since the manoeuvre involves an axial load, valgus and supination of the forearm. A similar situation occurs if the patient is asked to perform a press-up. The same forces are applied to the elbow and once more result in apprehension.[16] The patient is reluctant to extend the elbow fully (Figure 3.16).

Summary

Summary of elbow examination
Step 1   Stand the patient and look
Step 2   Move
Step 3   Feel
Step 4   Provocative tests
Step 5   Instability tests

Figure 3.16 Apprehension signs. The patient is reluctant to extend the elbow fully when rising from a chair and pushing up with his or her arms.

As with the wrist the sequence look, move, feel appears to flow better than the traditional look, feel, move.

Stand and look

Stand and look from the front, assessing the carrying angle. Look from the sides and then posteriorly and never forget to look medially, especially for any scars.

Move

With the shoulders abducted, ask the patient to extend both elbows and then to flex and compare the two, and ask him or her to put the elbows to the side and test for pronation and supination. This pronation or supination can be quantified by either asking the patient to hold a pencil in the hand or to point the thumb upwards and compare each side.

Feel

Knowing the anatomy of the structures being palpated is essential as the elbow is a superficial joint, therefore tenderness over a specific structure indicates pathology in that structure.

Put one finger on the medial epicondyle, one finger on the lateral epicondyle and one on the tip of the olecranon. Feel for medial tenderness and then flex and extend the elbow and feel for a subluxing ulnar nerve. Palpate the lateral epicondyle and feel for lateral tenderness and then rotate the forearm and feel for the radial head.

Feel for symmetry of the elbow by palpating these bony prominences. In extension normally these three bony prominences form a straight line but in 90° of flexion they form an isosceles triangle.

Finally, palpate the anterior structures, especially for the biceps tendon insertion.

Provocative tests

Provocative tests are then carried out, especially if the patient has medial or lateral tenderness.

If the patient has medial tenderness then the provocative test for golfer's elbow is performed. If the patient has lateral tenderness then the provocative test for tennis elbow is performed.

The provocative test for the medial side is performed by asking the patient to flex the wrist and prevent the examiner from straightening it. This results in increased pain in the region of the medial epicondyle.

A similar test is done for tennis elbow. Try to straighten an extended wrist against resistance. If this results in pain in the region of the lateral epicondyle then this is a positive provocative test for lateral epicondylitis.

Instability tests

Instability tests are for the medial collateral (valgus) and the lateral collateral (varus) ligaments.

Medial collateral

Stability is assessed by externally rotating the shoulder to lock it and by slightly flexing the elbow to unlock the elbow and providing a valgus force to the elbow.

Lateral collateral

The test for the lateral collateral ligament is performed by internally rotating the shoulder to lock it, slightly flexing the elbow to unlock it and providing a varus force.

Posterolateral rotatory instability

This is assessed by the pivot shift test. This is a painful test and is usually not required in the clinical exam. It is performed on a supine patient. The shoulder and elbow are both flexed to 90°. An axial force is applied to the supinated forearm. At the same time a valgus force is applied to the elbow. The resulting subluxation is reduced with a clunk as the elbow is extended towards 45°.

References

1 Andrews JR, Whiteside JA. Common elbow problems in the athlete. *J Orthop Sports Physiother* 1993;**6**:289–295.

2 Stanley D. Prevalence and aetiology of symptomatic elbow osteoarthritis. *J Shoulder Elbow Surg* 1994;**3**:386–389.

3 Morrey BF, Chow EY. Passive motion of the elbow joint. *J Bone Joint Surg (Am)* 1976;**58A**:501–508.

4 Yamamoto I, Ishii S, Usui M, Ogino T, Kaneda K. Cubitus varus deformity following supracondylar fracture of the humerus: a method for measuring rotational deformity. *Clin Orthop* 1985;**201**:179–185.

5 Major HP. Lawn tennis elbow. *BMJ* 1883;**ii**:557.

6 Mardam-Bey T, Ger E. Congenital radial head dislocation. *J Hand Surg* 1979;**4**:316–320.

7 Thompson H, Garcia A. Myositis ossificans: aftermath of elbow injuries. *Clin Orthop* 1967;**50**:129–134.

8   Baker BE, Bierwagen D. Rupture of the distal tendon of biceps brachii. *J Bone Joint Surg (Am)* 1985;**67A**:414–417.

9   Hartz CR, Linscheid RL, Gramse RR, Daube JR. The pronator teres syndrome: compressive neuropathy of the median nerve. *J Bone Joint Surg (Am)* 1981;**63A**:885–890.

10 Spinner M, Kaplan EP. The relationship of the ulnar nerve to the medial intermuscular septum in the arm and its clinical significance. *Hand* 1976;**8**:239–242.

11 Bennett BS. Triceps tendon rupture. *J Bone Joint Surg (Am)* 1962; **44A**: 741–744.

12 Nirschl RP. Elbow tendinosis/tennis elbow. *Clin Sports Med* 1992;**4**:851–870.

13 Regan WD, Korinek SL, Morrey BF, An KN. Biomechanical study of ligaments about the elbow joint. *Clin Orthop* 1991;**271**:271.

14 Jobe F, Elattrache N. Reconstruction of the MCL. In Morrey BF (ed) *Masters Techniques: The Elbow.* Philadelphia: Raven Press, 1994.

15 O'Driscoll SW, Bell DF, Morrey BF. Postero-lateral rotatory instability of the elbow. *J Bone Joint Surg (Am)* 1991;**73A**:440–446.

16 Regan WD, Morrey BF. Physical examination of the elbow. In Morrey BF (ed) *The Elbow and its Disorders*, 3rd edition. Philadelphia: WB Saunders, 2000.

Chapter

4

Examination of the wrist

Stephen Bostock

History

Patients with wrist problems often have a paucity of clinical signs. Specific provocative tests can be both difficult to perform and equivocal in their interpretation. A thorough history is therefore essential.

The history should start by recording the age, occupation and handedness of the patient, together with any affected recreational activities, including sports and hobbies.

The basic complaint needs to be established. Is it pain, weakness, a swelling, stiffness or a combination of these? Are there other symptoms? How long has there been a problem? Was there an injury or has the onset been insidious? What was the nature of the injury; was it a single event and, if so, did it receive treatment at the time?

The site and nature of *pain* should be established (Figure 4.1). The patient should be asked to try to localize it as accurately as possible (for example, by pointing). What is its nature; is it constant or intermittent, sharp, dull or 'burning'? Is it worse with use and eased by rest? Are there particular movements that aggravate the pain such as turning taps, opening jars?

Stiffness may be a part of the presenting problem. If so, which movements are restricted? Is there associated discomfort and how does this interfere with the use of the arm in functional terms?

Swelling may be present. Is this the main problem? Is it painless? Is the swelling growing or does its size vary?

Other symptoms may also be present; for example, a 'click' or a 'clunk'. If so, is it painful? Has there been an injury? Is the wrist *weak*? Does the weakness appear to be secondary to pain?

The history also needs to document the impact that the patient's wrist problem has had on activities of daily living, work, sports and other hobbies.

Examination

Inspection

The patient should be sat comfortably in a chair directly facing the examiner. Patients will usually offer their wrist forward in pronation (Figure 4.2). Observe this and then place the opposite side in a corresponding position with the elbows to the sides. Look carefully and systematically at the wrists. Look at the overall alignment and shape of the forearm, wrist and hand. Is there obvious deformity? What is the likely nature of this deformity (e.g. Madelung's deformity, rheumatoid arthritis, radial malunion)? Is there an obvious swelling in the wrist (dorsal wrist ganglion, carpal boss)?

Rheumatoid arthritis[1]

Features of rheumatoid arthritis are usually prominent around the wrist. These include:

- Extensor synovitis
- Extensor tendon rupture
- Dorsal subluxtion of the distal radioulnar joint (DRUJ)
- Volar subluxation and supination of the carpus
- Ulnar translocation of the carpus with radial metacarpal drift and ulnar drift of the fingers
- Flexor synovitis
- Flexor tendon rupture
- Finger deformities
- Bilaterality
- Other joint involvement.

Examination Techniques in Orthopaedics, Second Edition, ed. Nick Harris and Fazal Ali. Published by Cambridge University Press. © Cambridge University Press 2014.

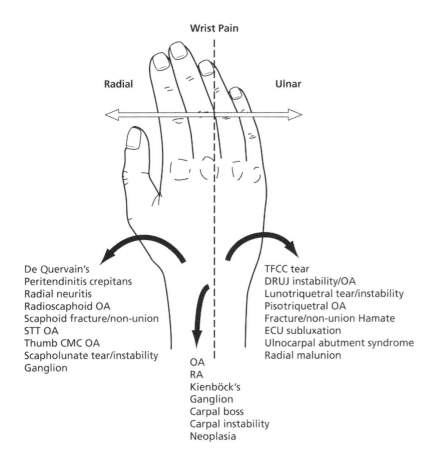

Wrist Pain

Radial

Ulnar

De Quervain's
Peritendinitis crepitans
Radial neuritis
Radioscaphoid OA
Scaphoid fracture/non-union
STT OA
Thumb CMC OA
Scapholunate tear/instability
Ganglion

OA
RA
Kienböck's
Ganglion
Carpal boss
Carpal instability
Neoplasia

TFCC tear
DRUJ instability/OA
Lunotriquetral tear/instability
Pisotriquetral OA
Fracture/non-union Hamate
ECU subluxation
Ulnocarpal abutment syndrome
Radial malunion

Figure 4.1 Line drawing illustrating sites of commonly occurring pathologies about the wrist. CMC, carpometacarpal; DRUJ, distal radioulnar joint; ECU, extensor carpi ulnaris; OA, osteoarthritis; RA, rheumatoid arthritis; STT, scaphotrapeziotrapezoid; TFCC, triangular fibrocartilage complex.

Radial malunion

Deformity most commonly follows the pattern of the original fracture; for example, radial shortening and prominence of the distal ulna.

Madelung's deformity[2]

This condition arises in childhood. There is volar bowing of the distal radius, with dorsal prominence of the distal ulna. Look for hypoplastic radius, family history, absence of trauma and bilaterality. (Dorsal bowing may occur and is described as 'reverse Madelung's deformity'.)

Dorsal wrist ganglion

Dorsal wrist ganglions usually arise from and overlie the scapholunate ligament[3] (just distal to Lister's tubercle). They will transilluminate if large. Pain without swelling in this area may represent an 'occult' ganglion.[4]

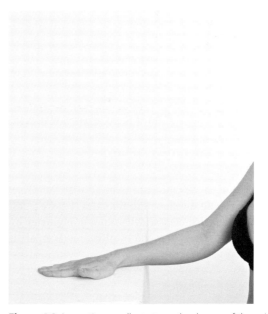

Figure 4.2 Inspection usually starts on the dorsum of the wrist.

Carpal boss[5]

A carpal boss is a bony hard swelling at the level of the second and third carpometacarpal (CMC) joints dorsally. These are more distal than most simple ganglia. To confuse matters there may be an associated small overlying ganglion.

Extensor digitorum brevis manus

This is an extra (vestigial) muscle whose presence distal to the extensor retinaculum may confuse it with a ganglion or extensor synovitis. It moves with finger extension.

Once the dorsum has been inspected, ask the patient to supinate. Is this movement pain-free or restricted?

Carefully inspect this side of the wrist from its ulnar aspect back to radial, thus completing the circumference. Look for scars and swelling, comparing right with left. A volar ganglion on the radial side must be examined with the underlying artery in mind using Allen's test (see Chapter 5).

Finally, fully flex the elbows and inspect the ulnar aspect of the wrists, looking at the profile of the distal ulna in relation to the radius. Asymmetry suggests possible DRUJ subluxation (dorsal or volar).

Range of motion

Flexion/extension

Extension can be assessed by placing the palms of the hands together and lifting up the elbows (this allows for direct comparison of the right and left sides). Flexion can be measured in a similar way, with the dorsum of both hands in apposition (Figures 4.3a, b). A goniometer may be used to quantify the range more accurately. Each wrist is measured in turn. For wrist extension the goniometer is placed on the volar aspect in line with the radius and third metacarpal. For flexion, the goniometer is placed dorsally in the same line.

Radial and ulnar deviation

Radial and ulnar deviation are assessed with the wrists in pronation and the elbows to the sides (Figure 4.3c). The range can also be assessed with a goniometer by alignment with the radius and the third metacarpal on the dorsum of the wrist.

Pronation and supination

This is assessed with the elbows to the sides (Figure 4.3d), again with a comparison of sides.

On occasions it may be appropriate to assess 'active' range of motion in addition to the passive measurements.

Palpation

Palpation should also follow a system. Work across the wrist, initially on its dorsal aspect and then volarly (Figure 4.4). Palpation should be aimed at specific anatomic landmarks.

Now examine the wrist area in more detail, starting on the dorsal aspect and working across from radial to ulnar. Is there fullness in the anatomical snuffbox? (Scaphoid pathology.) Does the area around the radial styloid and first extensor compartment look swollen? (De Quervain's disease.) Is there a swelling on the dorsum and, if so, what structure might this be overlying?

An attempt should be made to localize the area of tenderness as accurately as possible (Figure 4.5).

De Quervain's disease

This is characterized by swelling and pain localized to the first extensor compartment (radial styloid). Crepitus may be present ('wet leather sign'). There may be an associated ganglion.

Radial neuritis (Wartenberg's neuralgia)

Radial neuritis presents as pain and tenderness over the terminal cutaneous branches of the radial nerve. Look for a history of trauma.

Peritendinitis crepitans (intersection syndrome)[6]

This is bursitis between abductor pollicis longus (APL)/extensor pollicis brevis (EPB) and the wrist extensors (extensor carpi radialis longus [ECRL] and extensor carpi radialis brevis [ECRB]). Crepitus is often palpable together with tenderness. This area of discomfort is more proximal than that in De Quervain's disease.

Provocative and instability tests

A number of provocative tests for various conditions about the wrist have been described (Table 4.1). Clearly it would be inappropriate to perform all the available tests on every patient. Some sort of strategy is needed based on the history and examination thus far.

(a)

(b)

(c)

(d)

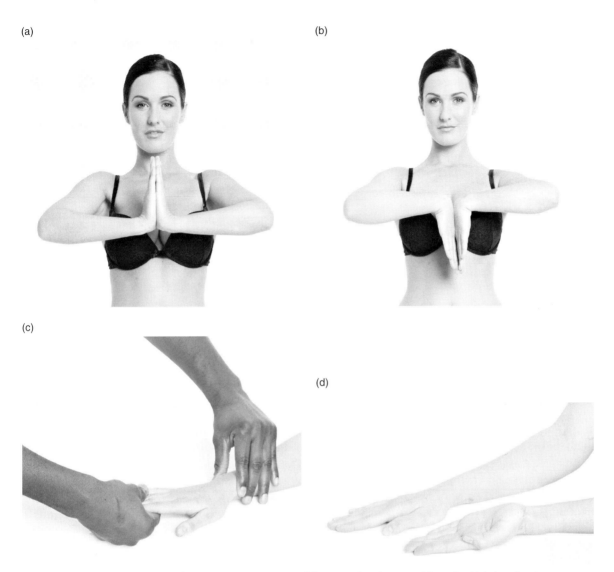

Figures 4.3 a and **b** A simple way of assessing wrist extension and flexion. **c** Ulnar deviation. **d** Pronation (right hand) and supination (left hand).

Finkelstein's test[7]

The examiner supports the forearm with one hand. With the other hand the thumb is adducted and the wrist ulnarly deviated to put tension on the APL and EPB tendons (Figure 4.6). A positive test will elicit pain over the inflamed area in the region of the radial styloid.

Carpal instability

A term that is used to describe a wide variety of pathological conditions, all of which stem from disruption of the complex ligament system that controls the relative motion of the bones that form the carpus.

Scapholunate instability

Rupture of the scapholunate ligament permits abnormal movement between the scaphoid and the lunate. Kirk Watson described a provocative test to reproduce and clinically detect this abnormal movement. This test is known variously as the 'Kirk Watson test', the 'Watson test', the 'scaphoid test' or the 'scaphoid shift'.[8] Two other tests for scapholunate instability are the 'scaphoid thrust' and the 'scaphoid lift' tests.[9,10]

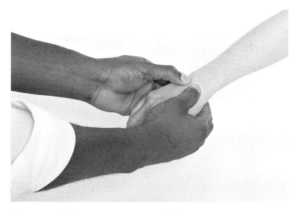

Figure 4.4 Palpating in sequence: the dorsal, volar, radial and ulnar aspects of the wrist.

Scaphoid shift test (Kirk Watson)[8]

The examiner uses one hand to grasp the wrist, placing the fingers dorsally (index or middle fingertips to lie over the area of the scapholunate ligament). The thumb is placed over the scaphoid tubercle volarly. With the examiner's other hand the patient's wrist is moved from ulnar into radial deviation whilst maintaining pressure on the scaphoid tubercle (Figures 4.7 and 4.8). With radial deviation the scaphoid will usually flex. The thumb pressure resists this and, in the presence of a scapholunate tear, the scaphoid subluxes dorsally off the radius. A positive test occurs when this abnormal movement is felt by the examiner, often as a 'click'. Pain may also be a significant finding, but is less specific for scapholunate instability. The scaphoid shift is positive in up to 36% of 'normal' individuals.[11]

Scaphoid thrust test[9]

Lane has described a modification of the Kirk Watson test which he originally, rather confusingly, named the scaphoid shift test, but which has been renamed the scaphoid thrust test. The patient's hand is held in the same way as for the scaphoid shift with the examiner's thumb over the scaphoid tubercle. The wrist is rocked backwards and forwards from radial to ulnar deviation until the patient is relaxed and guarding has been eliminated. The scaphoid tubercle is then quickly pressed by the examiner's thumb with the wrist in slight radial deviation and neutral flexion/extension. For a positive test the scaphoid should be felt to move dorsally.

Scaphoid lift test[10]

A third test has been described in which the lunate is stabilized with the thumb and index finger of one hand whilst the scaphoid is translocated volarly and dorsally using the other thumb and index finger.

> **Midcarpal instability**
>
> The 'drawer tests' may be positive in patients with midcarpal instability, although are more commonly an assessment of general ligamentous laxity. More specific tests for midcarpal instability are the 'midcarpal shift test' and the 'pivot shift test'.

Radiocarpal and midcarpal drawer tests

The examiner firmly grasps the patient's forearm with one hand. With the other hand the patient's hand is held at metacarpal level and a distracting force is applied. A dorsal and volar translating force is then applied and the amount of movement assessed (comparing sides). If the examiner then repeats the manoeuvre but moves his distal hand proximally to the level of the proximal carpal row, it has been suggested that it is possible to assess laxity across the midcarpal joint.

Midcarpal shift test[10,12]

The examiner stabilizes the forearm with one hand. With his other hand the examiner places his thumb over the capitate dorsally. A volarly directed force is applied as the wrist is ulnarly deviated. If there is a palpable 'clunk' as the wrist approaches full ulnar deviation then this is a positive test. The degree of laxity and clunking has been graded (I–V). It is thought that in patients with midcarpal instability the proximal carpal row is slow to dorsiflex as the wrist ulnarly deviates and that the clunk represents a catch-up movement.

A slight variation on this test applies an axial rather than a volar load as the wrist is ulnarly deviated.

Pivot shift test[13,14]

The elbow is placed on a firm surface and the hand is fully supinated. The forearm is held firmly. The hand is radially deviated and pressure applied to the dorsoulnar aspect of the carpus. The hand is then ulnarly deviated. A normal wrist 'notches' into a less supinated position as the capitate engages the lunate.

(a)

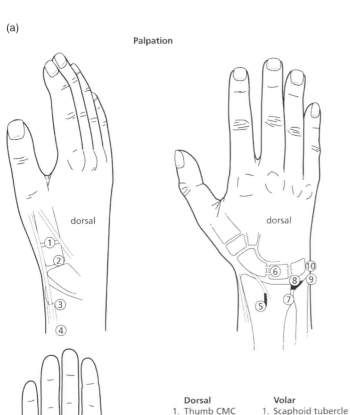

Palpation

Dorsal
1. Thumb CMC
2. ASB
3. Radial styloid
4. Distal radius
5. Lister's tubercle
6. SLL
7. DRUJ
8. TFCC
9. Ulnar styloid
10. Ulnar snuffbox

Volar
1. Scaphoid tubercle
2. Radial styloid
3. Radial artery
4. FCR
5. FCU
6. Pisiform
7. Hamate (hook)

Figure 4.5 a A systematic approach to palpation around the wrist. **b** Possible pathologies detectable by palpation over the radial aspect of the wrist. ASB, anatomical snuffbox; CMC, carpometacarpal; DRUJ, distal radioulnar joint; FCR, flexor carpi radialis; FCU, flexor carpi ulnaris; OA, osteoarthritis; SLL, scapholunate ligament; TFCC, triangular fibrocartilage complex.

(b)

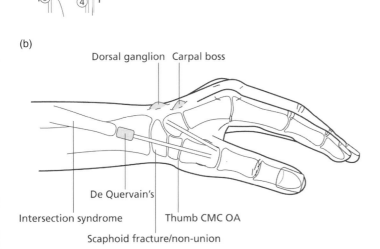

Dorsal ganglion   Carpal boss

De Quervain's

Intersection syndrome

Thumb CMC OA

Scaphoid fracture/non-union

Table 4.1 Provocative and instability tests

Condition	Test
De Quervain's	Finkelstein's
Scapholunate instability	Scaphoid shift (Kirk Watson)
	Scaphoid thrust
	Scaphoid lift
Midcarpal instability	Midcarpal shift
	Pivot shift
Lunotriquetral instability	Ballottment (Reagan)
	Shear
Ulnar-sided pathology	Ulnocarpal stress
Pisotriquetral arthritis	Grind
Distal radioulnar joint instability	Piano key
	Radioulnar drawer test
	Compression
	Dimple sign
Triangular fibrocartilage complex tear, extensor carpi ulnaris subluxation	Compression
Hamate fracture/ non-union	

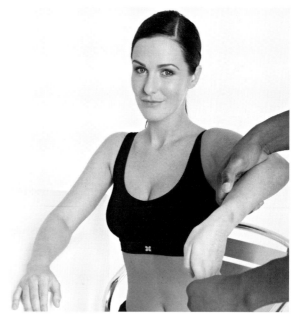

Figure 4.6 Finkelstein's test. This stresses the first extensor compartment and is a provocative test for De Quervain's tenosynovitis. The thumb is flexed followed by ulnar deviation of the wrist.

Ulnar-sided wrist pain

The diagnosis of ulnar-sided wrist pain is difficult. The 'ulnocarpal stress test'[15] is a general screening test for ulnar-sided pathology. More specific tests have been described to try and separate out the underlying pathology.

Difficulty arises not least because of the interrelationship between the different processes. For example, ulnocarpal abutment (also ulnar impaction[16]) may be associated with a triangular fibrocartilage complex (TFCC) tear. The TFCC is a stabilizer of the DRUJ and a tear may therefore be associated with painful instability of the DRUJ. Thus, in the context of clinical examination it may be impossible and inaccurate to try to establish a single diagnosis.[17]

Ulnocarpal stress test[15]

With the forearm supported the examiner applies axial load to the wrist, which is held in ulnar deviation

and neutral flexion/extension. The forearm is then rotated. A positive test elicits pain on the ulnar side of the wrist.

A variation of this test is to hold the forearm with the wrist in neutral pronation and supination but ulnar deviation. The wrist is then flexed and extended. A positive test elicits pain.

Lunotriquetral ligament injuries (instability)

Carpal instability associated with predominantly ulnar-sided symptoms may be secondary to a lunotriquetral ligament tear. Reagan et al. have described a ballottment test.[19] There are also compression and shear tests whilst three other tests have been described by Christodoulou and Bainbridge.[20]

Ballottment test (Reagan)[18]

The lunate is fixed between the thumb and index finger of one hand. With the other thumb and index finger the triquetrum (and pisiform) are displaced dorsally and volarly (Figure 4.9). Laxity, pain or crepitus indicates a positive result.

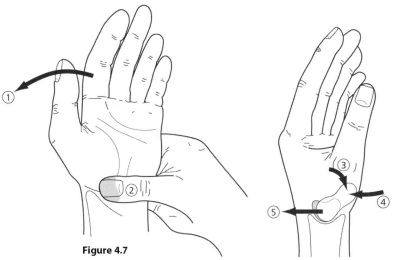

1. The wrist is moved from ulnar into radial deviation
2. Pressure is applied by the examiner's thumb to resist scaphoid flexion
3. Scaphoid rotates (flexes) with radial deviation of the wrist
4. Applied force (examiner's thumb)
5. Subluxation (may be felt by examiner's index/middle finger)

Figure 4.7

(a)

(b)

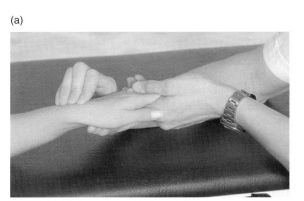

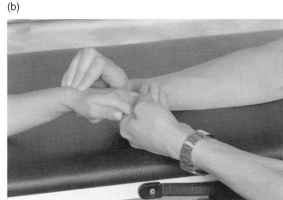

Figures 4.7 and 4.8 The scaphoid shift test (Kirk Watson). Pressure over the scaphoid tubercle with the examiner's thumb whilst radially deviating the wrist causes a click or pain in scapholunate instability.

Shear test

The lunate is stabilized with the thumb over the dorsal aspect of the wrist. A force is then applied to the pisiform volarly, thus indirectly applying a shear force across the lunotriquetral joint.

Chistodoulou and Bainbridge[19] describe three further tests for lunotriquetral instability. In the most commonly used of these the wrist is dorsiflexed, radially deviated and the forearm fully pronated. The examiner's thumb pushes against the pisiform whilst the fingers apply counterpressure over the distal ulna. Whilst this pressure is maintained the wrist is brought into a neutral position. A positive result elicits pain

and sometimes a click as the pisiform 'reduces' during this manoeuvre.

> **Pisotriquetral arthritis**
>
> *Pisotriquetral arthritis is a cause of ulnar-sided wrist pain. Many of the tests described for lunotriquetral tears apply compression across the pisotriquetral joint and these tests are likely to be positive for pain where there is arthritis. A grind test has also been described.*

Grind test

In this the pisiform is held between the thumb and index finger. Compression is applied and the pisiform is displaced back and forth in a radial and ulnar direction.

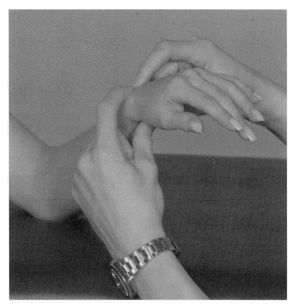

Figure 4.9 Ballottment test. Fixing the lunate between the finger and thumb of one hand and displacing the triquetrum dorsally and volarly with the other causes pain or demonstrates laxity in patients with lunotriquetral instability.

> ### The distal radioulnar joint
>
> *Problems with the DRUJ may be isolated or part of a complex of injuries. Pain on pronation and supination may be exacerbated by compression. The '(radioulnar) drawer test', 'piano key test' and 'dimple sign' may indicate joint subluxation.*

Compression test

Pain on pronation and supination of the forearm may not be specific to the DRUJ. The compression test applies a force across the joint by squeezing the forearm which is then pronated and supinated. A positive test occurs where this increases pain in the region of the DRUJ.

Piano key test

The examiner stabilizes the forearm distally with his fingers over the volar aspect. The thumb then presses over the distal ulna (Figure 4.10). Increased excursion suggests dorsal subluxation. (This test can be used to demonstrate caput ulnae seen in conditions such as rheumatoid arthritis.)

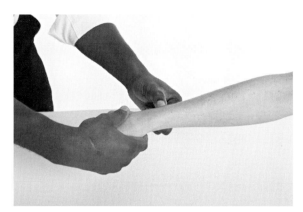

Figure 4.10 The piano key test. Pressure over the ulnar styloid by the examiner's thumb in a dorsal to volar direction will demonstrate increased excursion in patients with dorsal subluxation.

Radioulnar drawer test

The flexed elbow is rested on a firm surface. The radius is stabilized with one hand. The ulna is grasped between the fingers and thumb of the other hand and moved dorsally and volarly. This can be repeated with the forearm in different positions of pronation and supination and should be compared with the opposite side. Laxity of the DRUJ can be assessed and, if excessive, may be a sign of instability, especially if this is associated with discomfort.

Dimple sign

Longitudinal traction is applied across the wrist. A force is applied to the dorsal aspect of the ulnar shaft. If a 'dimple' appears at the level of the DRUJ then this suggests volar subluxation.

Triangular fibrocartilage complex tears

The diagnosis of TFCC tears may be suspected from tenderness in the hollow just distal to the ulnar head. This can be confirmed by the **TFCC compression test**. Here the patient's forearm is pronated and the elbow flexed. The examiner grasps the forearm with one hand and grasps the fingers with the other hand. The wrist is then loaded by compressing the hand proximally against the forearm. It is then moved in radial and ulnar directions. A painful click may indicate a TFCC tear (Figure 4.11).

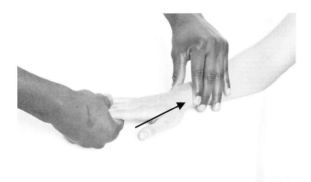

Figure 4.11 The TFCC compression test. Axial load across the wrist followed by radial and ulnar deviation will result in a painful click.

Extensor carpi ulnaris (ECU) subluxation

Subluxation of the ECU tendon may be provoked by placing the forearm in supination and ulnar deviation. With dorsiflexion the tendon may be painful and can sometimes be felt to sublux volarly.

Hamate fracture/non-union

Tenderness over the hook of the hamate (distal and radial to the pisiform) may indicate an underlying fracture or non-union. In these conditions the pain may be made worse by resisted flexion of the little and ring fingers with the wrist in ulnar deviation.

Overview of the upper limb

The wrist should not be considered in isolation. Some attention needs to be paid to the upper limb in general:

- The neurological status: Briefly assess motor and sensory function
- The neurological status: Palpate radial artery. Allen's test
- The neurological status: Briefly assess the shoulder, elbow and hand

Measurement of grip strength

Grip strength can be measured using a Jamar dynamometer. This provides an objective measurement of one aspect of hand function.

With the shoulder adducted and the elbow flexed to 90° the patient is asked to squeeze the dynamometer with maximum strength. The test is repeated three times for each wrist. A 'rapid exchange' technique has been described to detect submaximal effort.[20]

Summary

Summary of wrist examination
Step 1 Look
Step 2 Move
Step 3 Feel
Step 4 Special tests (depending on pathology detected in steps 1 to 3). These are both Provocative and Instability tests

As with the elbow the sequence look, move, feel appears to flow better than the traditional look, feel, move.

Look

Look at both palmar and dorsal aspects of the wrist.

Move

Dorsiflexion – hands together and lift both elbows up comparing sides

Palmarflexion – dorsum of hands together and move both elbows downwards

Radial and ulnar deviation

Pronation and supination, with elbows into side.

Feel

For tender areas (remember Lister's tubercle just proximal to scapholunate ligament).

Then, depending on tender area, this will direct you to perform the relevant special test.

Special tests – Provocative and instability tests

The following are the more commonly performed tests:

- Radial tenderness then perform Finkelstein's test
- Tenderness over the scapholunate ligament then perform Kirk Watson test
- Tenderness over lunotriquetral ligament then perform lunotriquetral ballottment test
- Tenderness over TFCC then perform TFCC compression test
- Prominence of the ulnar head then perform piano key test.

References

1   Wolfe SW (ed.) *Green's Operative Hand Surgery*, 6th edition. Edinburgh: Churchill Livingstone, 2010.

2   Schmidt-Rohlting B. *et al.* Madelung deformity: clinical features, therapy and results. *J Pediatr Orthop B* 2001;**10**:344–348.

3   Angelides AC, Wallace PF. The dorsal ganglion of the wrist: its pathogenesis, gross and microscopic anatomy, and surgical treatment. *J Hand Surg (Am)* 1976;**1**:228–235.

4   Sanders WE. The occult dorsal carpal ganglion. *J Hand Surg (Br)* 1985;**10B**:257–260.

5   The Carpal Boss. Review of diagnosis and treatment. *J Hand Surg (Am)* 2008;**33**:446–449.

6   Grundberg AB, Reagan DS. Pathological anatomy of the forearm: intersection syndrome. *J Hand Surg (Am)* 1985;**10**:299–302.

7   Finkelstein H. Stenosing tendovaginitis of the radial styloid process. *J Bone Joint Surg (Am)* 1930;**12A**:509–540.

8   Watson HK, Ashmead D, Makhlouf MV. Examination of the scaphoid. *J Hand Surg (Am)* 1988;**13A**:657–660.

9   Lane LB. The scaphoid shift test. *J Hand Surg (Am)* 1993; **18A**:366–368.

10 Cooney W (ed.) *The Wrist: Diagnosis and Operative Treatment*, 2nd edition. Philadelphia: Lippincott Williams & Wilkins, 2010.

11 Easterling KJ, Wolfe SW. Scaphoid shift in the uninjured wrist. *J Hand Surg (Am)* 1994; **19A**:604–606.

12 Feinstein WK, Lichtman DM, Noble PC, Alexander JW, Hipp JA. Quantitative assessment of the midcarpal shift test. *J Hand Surg (Am)* 1999;**24A**:977–983.

13 Tubiana R, Thomine J, Mackin E. *Examination of the Hand and Wrist*. London: Martin Dunitz, 1998.

14 Stanley J, Saffar P. *Wrist Arthroscopy*. London: Martin Dunitz, 1994.

15 Nakamura R, Horii E, Imaeda T, *et al.* The ulnocarpal stress test in the diagnosis of ulnar-sided wrist pain. *J Hand Surg (Br)* 1997; **22B**:719–723.

16 Sammer DM, Rizzo M. Ulnar impaction. *Hand Clin* 2010; **26**:549–557.

17 Sachar K. Ulnar sided wrist pain: evaluation and treatment of triangular fibrocartilage complex tears, ulnocarpal impaction syndrome, and lunotriquetral ligament tears. *J Hand Surg (Am)* 2008;**33**: 1669–1679.

18 Reagan DS, Linscheid RL, Dobyns JH. Lunotriquetral sprains. *J Hand Surg (Am)* 1984; **9A**:502–514.

19 Christodoulou L, Bainbridge LC. Clinical diagnosis of triquetrolunate ligament injuries. *J Hand Surg (Br)* 1999;**24B**: 598–600.

20 Hildreth DH, Breidenbach WC, Lister GD, Hodges AD. Detection of submaximal effort by use of the rapid exchange grip. *J Hand Surg (Am)* 1989;**14A**:742–745.

Examination of the hand

Joe A. Garcia

Examination of a patient's hand should always follow a comprehensive history. This provides valuable information to determine a diagnosis and to assess the impact that symptoms have on the patient's daily functions. Always remember to ask for hand dominance, occupation and recreational activities.

The following hand examination can confirm the working diagnosis or may raise possible alternative diagnoses. It may be used to assess a patient's hand function. Observations made from the history and examination may have an impact on the treatment options available.

There are numerous pathologies in the hand, which makes a standard approach helpful. By looking, feeling and assessing movement we can be sure of picking up most of the significant clinical findings. Special tests for individual pathologies may then complete the examination.

Screening

After exposing the upper limb adequately a *screening examination* is performed. Screening is an extremely important part of the examination, as close inspection whilst this is carried out will reveal clues to virtually all pathologies in the hand.

Look

First, inspect the hands with the palm facing upwards (Figure 5.1a). Then ask the patient to close the hands to make a fist (Figure 5.1b). Ask them to turn the hands over to face the floor and inspect the dorsum (Figure 5.1c). Again ask them to make a fist (Figure 5.1d). Lastly, ask the patient to flex the elbow and view the elbows, forearm and hands in profile (Figure 5.1e). Examine both hands together, as direct comparison between one and the other will help to reveal pathology.

The hand has a normal attitude, with a gradual cascade from one finger to another. An interruption in this cascade may result from many deformities. Some typical deformities may identify pathology simply on inspection.

Many other visual hints to pathology may be present: scars, diffuse and discrete swellings, muscle wasting, colour changes and nail deformities.

Feel for areas of tenderness or the characteristics of swellings.

Knowing the surface landmarks of the underlying anatomical structures is important when palpating areas of pathology. Focal points of tenderness will often point to an abnormality in the anatomical structure that you are palpating.

Move to assess the active and passive range of movement. These can be quantified by use of a goniometer (Figure 5.2).

The normal range of movements for the individual joints of fingers are:

- Distal interphalangeal joint (DIP): 0–80°
- Proximal interphalangeal (PIP) joint: 0–100°
- Metacarpal phalangeal (MCP) joint: 0–40° of hyperextension to 90° flexion.

For the individual joints of the thumb (Figure 5.3):

- Carpal metacarpal joint: contact with palm on adduction to 45° of abduction. Contact with palm to 60° of extension
- Metacarpal phalangeal joint: 10° of hyperextension to 55° of flexion
- Interphalangeal joint: 15° of hyperextension to 80° of flexion.

The *composite movements* of these joints allow the fingertips to touch the palm (Figure 5.4a). An inability to do this with one or more fingers suggests a

---

Examination Techniques in Orthopaedics, Second Edition, ed. Nick Harris and Fazal Ali. Published by Cambridge University Press. © Cambridge University Press 2014.

(a)

(b)

(c)

(d)

(e)

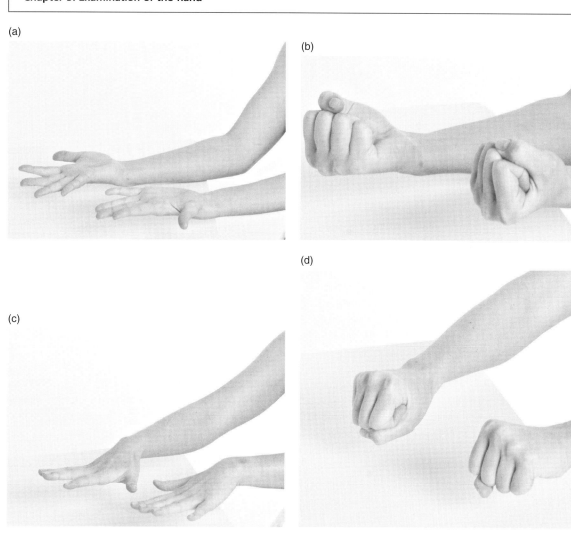

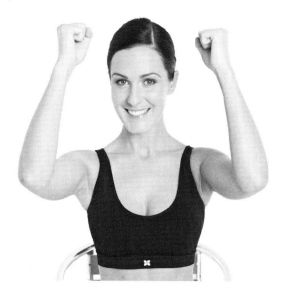

Figure 5.1 Screening for hand pathology. **a** Look at the hand, palms up. **b** Make a fist. **c** Look at the hand, palms down. **d** Make a fist. **e** Flex elbows and observe profile (hands closed and open).

(a)

(b)

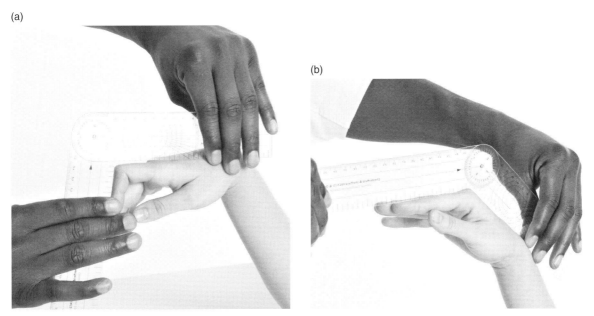

Figure 5.2 Measure the range of movements with a goniometer. **a** Proximal interphalangeal (PIP) joint. **b** Metacarpophalangeal (MCP) joint.

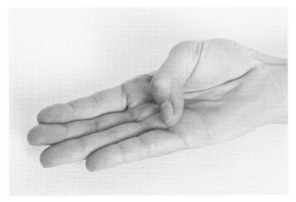

Figure 5.3 Range of thumb movements. Opposition is demonstrated here.

restriction in movement secondary to an underlying problem (Figure 5.4b). You can document the distance of the fingertip to the palm as a quick measure of movement loss.

Functions of hand

An *assessment of hand function* should be performed. Many decisions for surgery on the hand are based on function. This can be divided into grip/grasp strength (45% of function), pinch (45%), hook (5%) and paperweight (5%) (Figure 5.5). Hook refers to

lifting an object with the fingers flexed, e.g. carrying a shopping bag. Paperweight refers to resting the hand on an object. There are essentially three types of pinch: end (or pen) pinch, side (or key) pinch and chuck (tripod between thumb, index and middle fingers).

Assessment of joint deformities
Flexion contractures of the fingers

Flexion contractures of the small joints of the hand are a frequent problem. Their cause is multiple but the common outcome is poor hand function. Patients may have problems with work or sporting activities, but even simple day-to-day actions like putting hands in pockets or gloves may prove frustratingly difficult. The cosmetic appearance may also be a concern to the patient.

The patient's history may provide valuable information with regard to the aetiology. A history of injury to the hand or to the specific joint may be present. A history of multiple joint pathology may be consistent with an inflammatory arthropathy. A family history may be present in Dupuytren's disease.

Examination follows these principles.

Look: the initial observation should be meticulous and involves examining the hand in the different

(a)

(b)

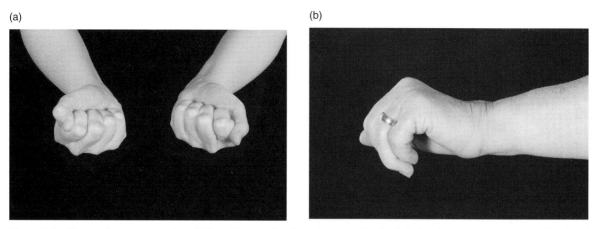

Figure 5.4 **a** Composite movements of small joints of fingers allow fingertips to touch palm. **b** Reduced composite movements of the hand because of arthritis.

(b)

(a)

(c)

(d)

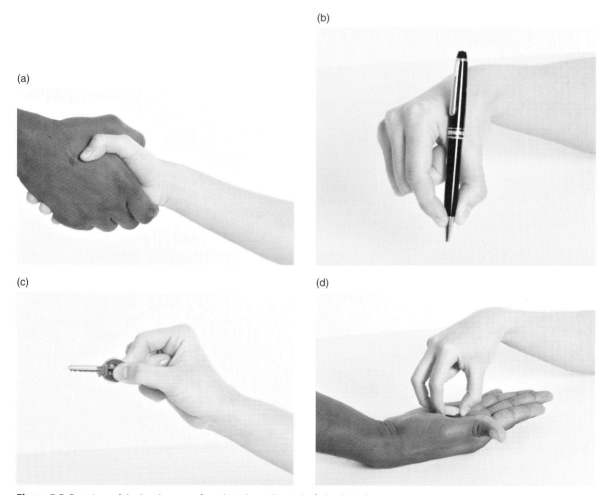

Figure 5.5 Functions of the hand: **a** grasp; **b** end pinch; **c** side pinch; **d** chuck pinch.

positions as described above in the screening test. From observations we should be able to describe:

a. Which finger or fingers are affected?
b. The degree of contracture at each affected joint – measure with goniometer for each affected joint.
c. Is there any obvious cause?
   i. Is there any scar tissue? This may arise from injuries and lacerations, incisions from operations and, occasionally, burns
   ii. Is there any abnormal tissue? The presence of Dupuytren's fibromatosis with nodules, cords and skin pitting may be seen on initial inspection
   iii. Is there swelling of the affected joint? Soft tissue or bony swelling may suggest an intrinsic problem of that joint.

Feel: previous observations will guide us to the specific parts of the hand that require careful palpation. If Dupuytren's disease is considered to be the cause, palpation determines the nature and extent of cords. Palpation can determine areas of tenderness around the joint that may be associated with an injury or a painful arthritis.

Move: is the contracture fixed? In other words, does the flexion contracture correct and by how much when it is passively straightened? Active and passive movements of the affected joints can be assessed. If there is a fixed flexion contracture it is still necessary to know how much flexion the patient has beyond the contracted position. If contractures are not fixed the range of passive extension can be measured. An extensor lag will highlight the active functional loss of the extensor mechanism, such as can occur with mallet injuries and flexible Boutonnières.

Specific pathologies causing a flexion deformity and their examination are described below.

Specific pathologies

Dupuytren's contracture of MCP/PIP (and, rarely, DIP) joints

In Dupuytren's disease the extent of the disease should be determined:

- Does it involve both hands?
- Which fingers and joints are involved?

The little finger is by far the commonest affected, at either the MCP or interphalangeal (IP) joints,

followed by ring and middle fingers and thumb (Figure 5.6).

When looking at obvious contractures the slightly less obvious problems may be missed. Pay attention to see if the thumb is involved, as cords in the first web space may lead to an adduction contracture. The fingers may also be adducted because of transverse ligament involvement.

A simple test to demonstrate contractures of the PIP and MCP joints is **Hueston's table top test.**[1] It may also be used as a guide for surgery. Ask the patient to place the palm of the hand flat on the table top. If there is a contracture of any of the PIP or MCP joints then the patient would be unable to perform this manoeuvre.

Assessing the condition of the skin is important. Look for and describe pitting and nodular formations. Severe contractures may lead to maceration of the skin. Any scars from previous surgery may affect your surgical decisions.

The skin condition may determine the need for dermofasciectomy and skin grafting.

An assessment of the subsequent loss of function is important. As in the rheumatoid hand, simple tests for hand function can be performed. Loss of ability to extend fingers and thumb so as to grasp may be very limiting.

If previous surgery has been performed then a digital Allen's test is important to assess the competency of both digital arteries.

Dupuytren's fibromatosis may be associated with other fibromatosis. Therefore, do not forget to exclude the presence of these, including Garrod's pads on the dorsal aspect of the PIP joint and nodules on the plantar aspect of feet (Ledderhose disease, 5% association). The patient may provide a history of penile involvement (Peyronie's disease, 3% association).

Multiple site fibromatosis, bilateral hand with multiple finger involvement, presence from a young age and a family history may suggest the presence of a Dupuytren's diathesis and may result in less rewarding surgical intervention with a higher risk of recurrence.

Flexion contractures of PIP joints secondary to a previous ligamentous injury

The PIP joint is stabilized by the collateral ligaments, accessory collateral ligaments and the volar plate. Injuries to the collateral ligaments or to the

(a)

(b)

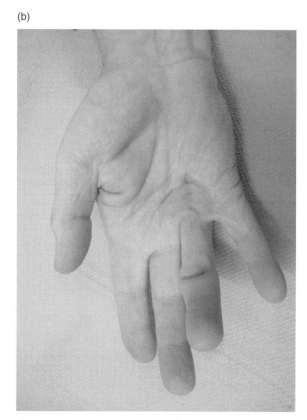

Figure 5.6 **a** Dupuytren's disease involving the abductor digiti minimi and the lateral sheet of finger. Note that the profile of the finger shows the deformity most clearly. **b** Dupuytren's disease leading to a pretendinous cord affecting the ring finger.

volar plate may lead to contractures resulting from scarring of these structures. These tend to occur particularly where these injuries are neglected or treated inappropriately. Even when treatment is appropriate, a gradual and progressive flexion contracture can occur.

It is also possible for hand injuries not directly involving the PIP joint to have similar consequences. Traumatic swelling or oedema of the hand can lead to PIP flexion contractures as fibrosis ensues. For this reason, it is important for these joints to be protected in a POSI (position of safety intrinsic) splint.

These flexion contractures are characteristically fixed and isolated to the PIP joint only. The degree of contracture can vary from mild to severe. There are no nodules or scarring to be seen or palpated. Some tenderness may be found on the palmar aspect over the volar plate and along the collateral ligaments, particularly if it is soon after the injury.

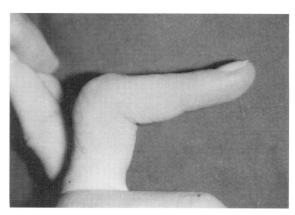

Figure 5.7 Boutonnière deformity with synovial proliferation on the dorsal aspect of the PIP joint.

Boutonnière deformity

This is a flexion deformity of a finger PIP joint with a secondary hyperextension of the DIP joint (Figure 5.7). It occurs as a result of an injury to the central slip of the extensor mechanism.

(a)

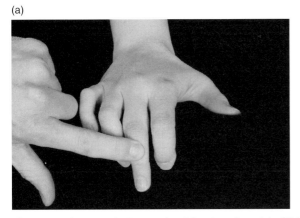

(b)

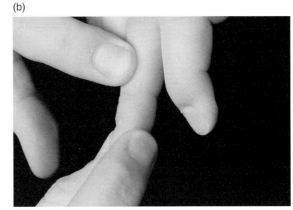

Figure 5.8 Elson's test for Boutonnière deformity. **a** Extend the PIP joint against resistance. **b** Weakness of extension of the PIP joint with hyperextension of the DIP joint indicates central slip rupture.

Damage of the central slip can occur as a result of a direct injury from sharp or blunt trauma. This results in a laceration or avulsion of the central slip. It may also occur following synovial proliferation in the dorsal aspect of the PIP joint in inflammatory arthropathies.

As a result the head of the proximal phalanx button-holes (Boutonnière) through these damaged tissues, leading to the PIP flexion deformity. The typical deformity includes extension of the DIP joint because, as the central slip tears or stretches, the two lateral bands displace in a palmar direction, producing further flexion of the PIP joint and secondary extension of the DIP joint.

Elson's test may be used to assess the presence of a competent central slip.[2] Place the hand flat on a table with the PIP joints at the edge of the table. Flex the PIP joint over the edge of the table. Ask the patient to actively extend against resistance (Figure 5.8a). Weakness of extension at the PIP joint with hyperextension of the DIP joint will occur when the central slip is ruptured (Figure 5.8b).

Mallet finger

This is a flexion deformity of the DIP joint. It occurs following an injury to the lateral slips. A laceration may occur proximal to the insertion or the tendon may be avulsed from the distal phalanx. This may be an intra-substance avulsion or may involve an avulsed fragment of bone.

The resulting consequence is an inability to extend the DIP joint. Inspection following the injury will identify an extensor lag. However much a patient

tries, he or she is unable to extend the joint actively. The joint may be passively correctable by the clinician but the corrected position will not be maintained when the pressure is released. If the injury is chronic it is possible for the deformity to become fixed, at which point it is no longer passively correctable. Determining these facts will guide what treatment options are available to the patient.

Intrinsic tightness leading to flexion contracture of the MCP joint

The intrinsic muscles include the dorsal and palmar interossei and the lumbrical muscles. The intrinsic muscles work through the extensor mechanism and by their direct attachment to the base of the proximal phalanx. Their actions through these insertions are to flex the MCP joint and extend the PIP and DIP joints.

As a result of scarring following injury or increased tone from a neurological problem the shortening of these structures leads to a fixed flexion deformity of the MCP joint and extension or decreased flexion of the IP joints.

Intrinsic tightness can be assessed by **Bunnell's test**. This assesses PIP joint flexion in two positions:

- With the MCP joint flexed (Figure 5.9a) – this will relax the tight intrinsic muscles and allow greater passive flexion of the PIP joint.
- Then, with the MCP joint extended (Figure 5.9b) – this will tighten the already tight intrinsic muscle and will reduce the passive flexion of the PIP joint.

In the normal hand passive flexion will be the same in all positions of the MCP joint.[3]

(a)

(b)

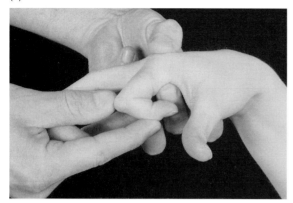

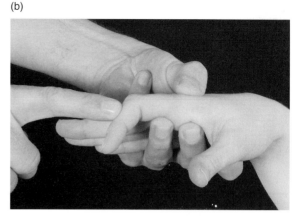

Figure 5.9 Bunnell's test. **a** Assess PIP joint flexion with the MCP joint flexed, then **b** compare the PIP joint flexion with the MCP joint extended.

Arthropathies of the hand

Patients with joint arthropathies present with pain, swelling and loss of movement. Deformities such as flexion contractures may also be part of these arthritic conditions. The aetiology may be degenerative, inflammatory or post-traumatic.

Degenerative arthropathies of the hand

First carpal metacarpal (CMC) joint arthritis

Arthritis at the base of the thumb is one of the commonest arthritic conditions in the hand. It presents with pain at the base of the thumb, extending into the thumb and sometimes proximally along the radial aspect of the wrist. Associated symptoms include a reduction in the range of movement and weakness in many functions of daily activity. Any movement involving grasping and gripping is painful and feels weak. The patient may also notice and complain of a deformity involving the thumb.

On examination, initial inspection may reveal a characteristic deformity of the thumb (Figure 5.10). This is:

1. A prominent base of thumb
   - May be described as 'squaring'.
2. An adduction deformity of the thumb metacarpal
   - Thumb in palm appearance.
3. A secondary hyperextension of the MCP joint.

The pathogenesis of this deformity starts with first CMC joint subluxation. The prominence at the base

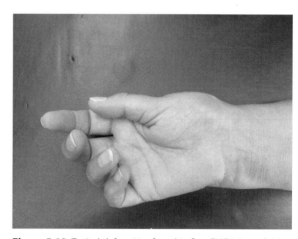

Figure 5.10 Typical deformities found in first CMC joint arthritis.

of the thumb results from the partially dorsally subluxed metacarpal base. There may also be soft tissue swelling from the damaged joint. The subluxed base of the metacarpal leads to metacarpal adduction. As the patient attempts to compensate for this to create a span across the first web space, there is a secondary hyperextension of the MCP joint.

The first CMC joint can be assessed further by asking the patient to actively move the thumb into extension, flexion, adduction and abduction. Note and measure any restriction in active movement and whether this reproduces pain. Measurement may be a simple comparison to the uninvolved side. Passive movement of the first CMC joint may again demonstrate these restrictions in movement and reproduce pain.

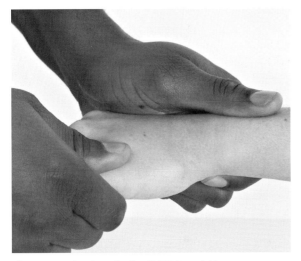

Figure 5.11 Grind test for first CMC joint arthritis.

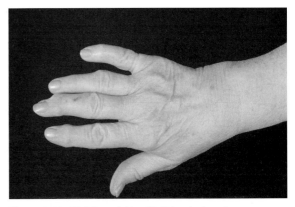

Figure 5.12 DIP joint arthritis with Heberden's nodes.

Palpation of the affected area may be commenced away from the problematic area. Palpation from distal to proximal along the thumb may reassure the patient. Arthritis in this joint frequently starts on the palmar half and the inflamed adjacent joint capsule is tender to palpation here. Therefore, in the earliest stages tenderness may be most pronounced on the palmar aspect of the joint, palpating at the base of the thenar eminence. In established arthritis, tenderness is present all around the joint and can be elicited directly over the dorsum of the joint.

To confirm clinical suspicions, special specific tests may be performed.

The **grind test**: this involves rotation of the metacarpal base against the trapezium (Figure 5.11). By holding the trapezium, compression against the scaphotrapeziotrapezoidal (STT) joint and scaphoid can be prevented. Any pain must therefore be originating in the first CMC joint. If there is no pain, releasing the trapezium will allow transfer of the force to the more proximal structures. Increased pain at that point will suggest pain from the STT joint (arthritis) or even more proximally from a scaphoid pathology (fracture or non-union).

DIP joint arthritis

Arthritis in these small joints is very common but is fortunately not always symptomatic. Patients will present with pain, stiffness and deformities.

Examination will identify the deformities and bony and soft tissue swellings. There may be a fixed flexion deformity of the joint because of the articular

degeneration. Often there is a lateral deformity, more in an ulnar direction, because of the radial forces applied to the fingertips. Osteophyte formation gives the typical bony swellings described as Heberden's nodes on either side of the midline (Figure 5.12). Soft tissue swelling may be diffuse because of an inflamed joint or more localized as a result of a mucoid cyst.

A mucoid cyst is a ganglion cyst arising from the joint and lying dorsally, often distal to the joint. Here, it may affect the nail bed and lead to ridging of the nail plate. Mucoid cysts may be present without an obviously arthritic joint. Palpation will reveal a tender joint and movements may be significantly restricted.

PIP joint arthritis

Arthritis in these joints is common and often symptomatic. Patients will present with pain, stiffness and deformities. Examination will identify the deformities and bony and soft tissue swellings.

There may be a fixed flexion deformity of the joint because of the articular degeneration. Osteophyte formation gives the typical bony swellings described as Bouchard's nodes on either side of the midline. Soft tissue swelling may be diffuse because of an inflamed joint. Range of movement may be restricted, more severely with chronic problems.

Inflammatory arthropathies of the hand
Rheumatoid arthritis

Examination of the rheumatoid hand should start by identifying the general features that allow consideration of this condition as a potential diagnosis.[4] This

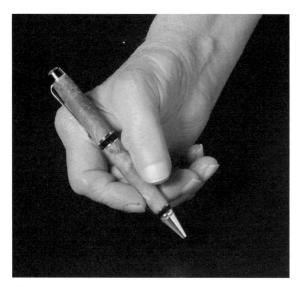

Figure 5.13 End (pen) pinch in a rheumatoid hand.

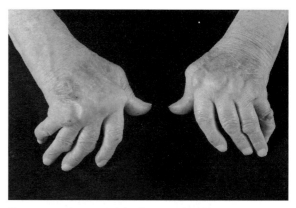

Figure 5.14 Overview of the rheumatoid hand.

includes the presence of a polyarticular, symmetrical arthropathy affecting the upper limbs, lower limbs and spine. Following general observations, the most significant abnormalities are examined and documented. The combination of these abnormalities may lead to functional problems with many activities of daily living. A simple assessment of function may be carried out with some 'consulting room' tests during the examination (Figures 5.5 and 5.13).

The examination of the hand starts with careful inspection. Look at the hand along with the rest of the upper limb, with hands palm down, facing upwards and then in profile. This will give a good overview of the condition of the upper limb. It will expose the proximal forearm and elbow and any rheumatoid nodules that may be present in this region. It may also expose any restriction in the range of movement in the shoulder and elbow.

Any abnormalities that have been noted can then guide the next stage of the examination to assess the individual joints or soft tissue pathologies present sequentially (Figure 5.14).

Wrist

In itself the wrist can be the site of considerable pain, leading to functional problems. But, even when there is minimal pain, significant deformities of the wrist can have an impact on the small joints of the hand. Assessing the condition of the rheumatoid wrist is therefore particularly important when there are other

hand deformities. The typical wrist deformity is radial deviation with volar subluxation and ulnar translation. Radial deviation of the carpal and metacarpal bones leads to changes in direction of pull of the flexor and extensor tendons. This contributes to the factors resulting in ulnar drift at the MCP joints. Any surgery to the MCP joints requires these problems being addressed to obtain a stable well orientated wrist.

Distal radial ulna joint (DRUJ)

The rheumatoid process that affects this joint leads to destruction of the soft tissue stabilizers of the joint, resulting in dorsal subluxation of the distal ulna. The subsequent prominence is called a caput ulna. The presence of a caput ulna should be noted as it may predispose to attritional damage of the extensor tendons. This, in combination with dorsal tenosynovitis, is a typical clinical sign found in a Vaughan-Jackson syndrome (see below).

MCP joint

The typical deformity is volar subluxation with ulnar drift.

MCP joint deformities in the hand are caused by a combination of pathologies:

- Radial deviation of the wrist and metacarpals
- Articular destruction
- Synovitis damaging the collateral ligaments and volar plates
- Stretching of the sagittal bands on the radial side and subsequent ulnar subluxation of the extensor tendons
- Intrinsic tightness.

On examination it may be possible to identify the presence of some of these problems with simple

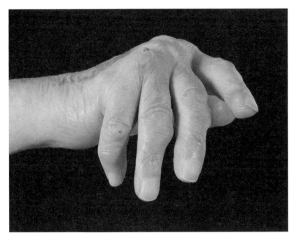

Figure 5.15 MCP joint deformities of the hand.

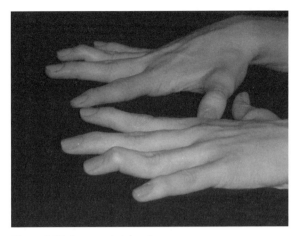

Figure 5.16 Swan neck deformity.

inspection (Figure 5.15). It can then be determined whether the MCP joints are reducible. Chronic subluxed joints cannot be reduced because of secondary changes. If they can be reduced, assess whether this reduction can be held temporarily. This gives an idea about the integrity of the extensor tendons. The relocation of the extensor tendon onto the dorsum of the metacarpal head may maintain the joint in a more normal position for a small period of time. Subsequent re-subluxation may also be seen. If this is absent, question whether the tendon has been ruptured.

Fingers – Boutonnière deformity

If the dorsal extensor tendon structures, such as the central slip, are destroyed by rheumatoid disease the PIP joint subluxes dorsally, resulting in PIP joint flexion. The lateral slips may secondarily collapse volarly, leading to an increased flexion force to the PIP joint and hyperextension of the DIP joint.

Staging is according to severity:[5]

- Stage 1 – mild extensor lag of 10–15° and the PIP joint is passively correctable. On passive PIP joint extension, DIP joint flexion becomes limited
- Stage 2 – more severe extensor lag of 30–40° but it is still passively correctable. There is no DIP joint flexion with correction
- Stage 3 – there is a fixed deformity of the PIP joint.

Fingers – swan neck deformity

If the volar plate and associated structures are damaged and attenuated by rheumatoid disease the PIP joint may hyperextend. Subsequently, a secondary

DIP joint flexion occurs from muscle imbalance (Figure 5.16).

A classification system is based around the mobility of the PIP joint:[6]

- Type I – PIP joint flexible in all positions
- Type II – PIP joint flexibility is affected by the presence of intrinsic tightness. Bunnell's test will demonstrate decreased flexibility with MCP joint extended compared to increased flexibility with MCP joint flexed
- Type III – PIP joint has limited flexibility in all positions and X-rays show a well preserved joint
- Type IV – PIP joint has limited flexibility in all positions but X-rays show joint destruction.

Thumb deformities

Deformities may be present at the first CMC joint, MCP joint and IP joint (Figure 5.17).

The typical patterns of deformity were described by Nalebuff: [7]

- Type I – Boutonnière deformity. Damage to the extensor tendon mechanism leads to dorsal subluxation of the MCP joint with secondary hyperextension of the IP joint (most common)
- Type II – type I deformity with additional subluxation of the first CMC joint
- Type III – swan neck deformity. Subluxation of the first CMC joint with adduction of the metacarpal leading to secondary hyperextension of the MCP joint and flexion of the IP joint
- Type IV – gamekeeper's thumb. Instability from laxity of the ulna collateral ligament of the MCP joint

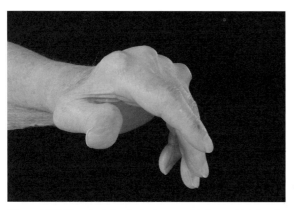

Figure 5.17 Thumb deformity in rheumatoid disease. Z-deformity consists of hyperextension at the IP joint and fixed flexion/subluxation at the MCP joint.

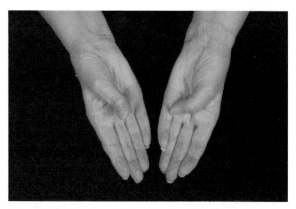

Figure 5.18 FPL rupture of the right thumb. Evident with the patient being asked to flex her thumb across the palm.

- Type V – volar plate damage leads to hyperextension of the MCP joint with secondary flexion of the IP joint, but differs from type III as there is no adduction of the metacarpal from first CMC joint dislocation.

Tendons

Tenosynovitis involving extensor tendon or flexor tendon sheaths — Rheumatoid disease may affect the synovial sheaths of flexor and extensor tendons. This will lead to swelling around the tendons, hampering their movements, causing damage to the tendon and potentially leading to complete ruptures.

Flexor tendon ruptures — **Mannerfelt lesion** – flexor pollicis longus (FPL) rupture (Figure 5.18).[8] This occurs as a result of attritional damage to the FPL around the distal pole of the scaphoid. Irregularities here are caused by wrist capsule synovitis and joint destruction.

If the rheumatoid process has not destroyed the IP joint, then active movement is lost but the IP joint will flex passively. A destroyed joint will have both passive and active loss of movement and will be more difficult to assess.

The differential diagnosis for an FPL rupture is:

- A triggering thumb: the thumb is unable to flex because the FPL is scarred down within the flexor sheath
- An anterior interosseous nerve (AIN) injury: an AIN palsy can be differentially assessed with index finger flexor digitorum profundus (FDP) function. Absence of active index finger DIP

joint flexion in combination with loss of thumb IP joint flexion may suggest an AIN palsy (OK sign).

The **tenodesis effect** may also be used to assess whether a tendon is intact. If the tendon is in continuity and attached to the distal phalanx, extending the wrist and thumb proximal to the IP joint should result in IP joint flexion. In a ruptured FPL, the joint will not flex. Compare one side to the other.

Extensor tendon rupture — As described previously, tenosynovitis around the extensor tendons and a caput ulna resulting from rheumatoid disease can ultimately lead to rupture of the extensor tendons (Figure 5.19).[9] The little finger is the first and most commonly involved. Sequential ruptures of the ring and middle fingers can then occur; this is Vaughan-Jackson syndrome.

The clinical features include an extensor lag of one or more fingers in the presence of dorsal tenosynovitis and a caput ulna. The latter two are not a must.

Extensor tendon rupture needs to be differentiated from:

1. MCP joint dislocation or subluxation. Passive extension may reduce the joint, at which point the extensor tendons can function and retain extension until the joint subluxes once again. If there is a fixed deformity, with no passive correction, then one can assume that it is an intrinsic joint problem.
2. Subluxation of the extensor tendon caused by sagittal band rupture or stretching. If the joint is not subluxed and the extensor lag is corrected passively,

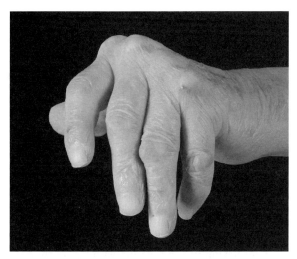

Figure 5.19 Extensor tendon rupture of left ring finger (Vaughan-Jackson syndrome). Note the synovitis on the dorsal region of the wrist.

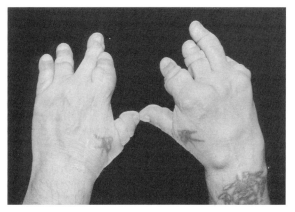

Figure 5.20 Collapsed skeleton of arthritis mutilans.

the extensor tendon may reduce onto the apex of the metacarpal head. While here it will maintain extension, but if it subluxes ulnarly because of a deficient sagittal band, the extensor lag will return. This subluxation may be seen or felt.

3. Posterior interosseous nerve palsy. All the fingers will be affected, as well as the thumb. There may also be weakness in wrist extension. Tenodesis effect will show tendons are intact.

If you have determined the presence of an extensor tendon rupture check for the presence of extensor indicis proprius (EIP), as this may be an option for reconstructive surgery. (See extensor pollicis longus (EPL) rupture.)

Rheumatoid nodules

Rheumatoid nodules occur usually on the extensor surface of the arm, including the olecranon, ulnar border of the forearm and over the IP joint of the fingers. They are the most common extra-articular manifestation of rheumatoid arthritis and are usually associated with aggressive disease.

Psoriatic arthritis

Psoriatic arthritis is a chronic inflammatory arthritis that develops in at least 5% of patients with psoriasis. The differentiating features include distal joint involvement and arthritis mutilans (mutilans may less commonly be seen in rheumatoid arthritis). Although DIP joint involvement is considered to be a classic and unique symptom of psoriatic arthritis, it occurs in only 5–10% of patients. Mutilans is a rare form of psoriatic arthritis, being found in 1–5% of patients[10] (Figure 5.20). In this severe arthritis there are radiographic changes of bone resorption, with dissolution of the joint. This gives rise to the typical 'pencil-in-cup' appearance.

On initial inspection psoriatic nail pitting may be seen. Psoriatic arthritis may be present with or without obvious skin lesions. Minimal skin involvement may be hidden (e.g. scalp, umbilicus, intergluteal cleft).

By looking at the arm in profile psoriatic plaques on the back of the elbow may be identified. Dactylitis with sausage digits is seen in as many as 35% of patients. With bone resorption and destruction severe deformities of the joints occur. Overlying skin may be redundant and a telescoping motion of the joint is possible.

Tendon problems
Extensor pollicis longus (EPL)

Patients with EPL ruptures present with problems using their thumb in day-to-day activities.[11] They have difficulties in abducting and extending their thumb. When combined this may be described as retropulsion. This inability leads to functional problems, as this is a requirement prior to grasping and gripping.

EPL ruptures occur suddenly, but a history of an underlying causal pathology must be investigated.

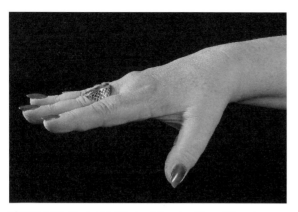

Figure 5.21 Abnormal attitude of thumb with an EPL rupture.

Synovitis secondary to an inflammatory arthritis such as rheumatoid may be present. A distal radial fracture in the recent past, even if not significantly displaced, may be the cause. If a radial fracture has been fixed with either volar or dorsal plates, prominent metalwork may be the culprit.

On examination, look for the attitude of the thumb; normally the thumb is held slightly abducted. With an EPL rupture it may lie in a slightly adducted position. The distal phalanx may lie in flexion, but this is not always the case. The extensor pollicis brevis (EPB) may work through the sagittal hood to maintain extension of the DIP joint.

Look for signs of an underlying cause of the EPL rupture; this could be inflammatory arthropathies and tenosynovitis. Also seek signs of a distal radial fracture, a malunion or scars from surgical intervention. A dorsal approach to fixation may result in metalwork being placed directly under EPL. A volar approach does not exclude metalwork protruding and damaging EPL. Screws and pegs from the volar side may be too long and prominent.

On palpation this metalwork may be prominent, palpable and tender. Synovitis along the course of the tendon may feel boggy and tender.

Ask the patient to perform a retropulsion movement and compare to the normal hand. Retropulsion is elevation of the thumb in an extended position and isolates the action of EPL, excluding EPB's action. A loss of EPL prevents the ability to perform this action (Figure 5.21).

When a diagnosis has been made, it is then necessary to consider the management options. One of the options available is surgical reconstruction with extensor indicis proprius (EIP). It is therefore

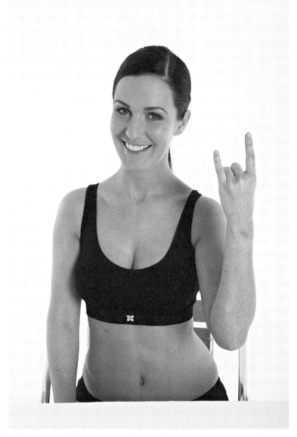

Figure 5.22 The presence of EIP and EDM can be tested for by flexing the other fingers in order to defunction EDC.

necessary to determine whether this is present as this is the tendon transfer of choice.[12]

The technique for **assessment of the presence of an EIP tendon** is to flex the MCP joints of all other fingers. This will defunction extensor digitorum communis (EDC). Any extension of the index finger MCP joint must therefore be the result of a present EIP. This may also be performed to assess the presence of extensor digiti minimi (EDM) (Figure 5.22).

Flexor digitorum profundus (FDP) and superficialis (FDS)

Loss of FDP or FDS function may occur from a direct injury or from tendon adhesions secondary to an injury, surgery, inflammatory synovitis or infection. With delayed presentation, patients may complain of loss of active movement or that the finger lies in an abnormal position.

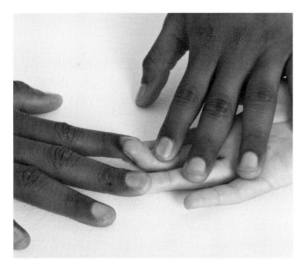

Figure 5.23 Testing FDP function.

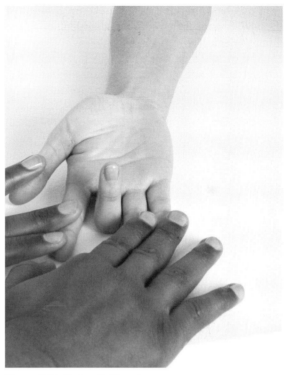

Figure 5.24 Testing FDS function.

Examination starts with inspection, which will provide clues to the underlying problem. Attention should be paid to the normal cascade of the fingers from both the dorsal and palmar aspect. If there is a break in the cascade then this suggests the possibility of a tendon injury.

Look for any obvious signs as to the cause of the FDP or FDS injury. Scars along the finger, palm and forearm may suggest a laceration or an operation in the past. Swellings or a thickness along the course of the tendon may point towards the location of the terminal stump of the tendon. It may also be the location of scarring of the tendon to adjacent tissues such as the sheath.

On palpation scarring may be felt as thickening along the flexor tendon sheath and in the palm. An ongoing inflammatory process may be tender.

Assessing movement is all about isolating the tendon to be tested and determining whether and to what extent it is working. **To test FDP**, isolate the DIP joint by holding the PIP joint in extension and asking the patient to flex at the DIP joint (Figure 5.23). Assess the strength with resistance against flexion. Compare to the other joints.

To test FDS (Figure 5.24), FDP needs to be excluded from the possibility that it may act upon and flex the PIP joint. As the FDP tendons have a common belly, the FDP can be prevented from contracting by holding all the fingers other than the finger being tested, with the DIP joints in extension. This prevents FDP flexing the finger

being tested. The only movement that will occur will be flexion of the PIP joint if the FDS is intact. The distal phalanx will not move and, in fact, remains quite floppy. If the FDS is absent then PIP joint flexion will not occur.

Quadrigia effect

When one FDP tendon is anchored down for any reason (adhesion, scarring, bony injury) it will impact on the ability of the other FDP tendons to contract because they all share a common muscle belly. This leads to loss of flexion of the remaining fingers.

Lumbrical plus

The characteristic feature of this problem occurs when attempting *active flexion* of a finger. In the lumbrical plus finger, active flexion of the MCP joint results in paradoxical extension of the PIP joint. It occurs when the FDP tendon is damaged distal to the origin of the lumbrical muscle on the FDP. This may be because of a divided tendon or one that has been repaired with a graft that is too long. Division of the tendon may be the result of an amputation of the distal phalanx.

In these situations the FDP tendon retracts proximally, taking with it the origin of the lumbrical muscle. When flexing the fingers, active contraction of the FDP tightens the lumbrical further. The action of the lumbrical through its insertion to the radial side of the lateral band is to extend the PIP joint. Passive flexion of the MCP joint will not give rise to the same problem.

Intrinsic minus and intrinsic plus

Intrinsic minus position is similar to a claw hand and is therefore seen in ulnar/median nerve injuries or Volkmann's ischaemic contracture. This is characterized by MCP joint hyperextension and IP joint flexion as a result of an imbalance of forces across these joints.

The intrinsic plus hand is caused by intrinsic tightness (see section on intrinsic tightness above). The typical position of the hand is MCP joint flexion and IP joint extension.

Trigger finger/thumb

This is a constriction of the flexor tendon by narrowing of the flexor tendon sheath A1 pulley. Patients complain of a very characteristic symptom. The finger gets stuck with the PIP joint flexed (IP joint of the thumb). It may spontaneously reduce with voluntary extension with the sensation of a sharp movement and click. With more severe disease the patient may need to reduce the finger with the other hand, forcing it into extension. The same sharp snapping sensation and click may be felt. This may also be painful. In the most severe cases the finger may be locked in flexion and may be impossible to reduce without surgery. The previous history of intermittent locking would point towards this most severe form of triggering rather than a fixed flexion deformity secondary to other causes. With even the early stages some, though not all, patients have significant levels of pain extending from the palm into the finger.[13]

Observation may identify the snapping of the finger from the flexed position back into extension. If a finger is placed over the A1 pulley, a thickening or nodule may be palpated, which moves suddenly on reduction of the finger. This nodule may be tender

and the tenderness may extend along the flexor tendon sheath distally.

Multiple trigger fingers may occur (exclude diabetes in these situations) and all the fingers should be assessed during the consultation. Trigger thumb is a similar process to that which results from the FPL catching at the entrance of its flexor tendon sheath, resulting in clicking or locking of the IP joint of the thumb.

Flexor tendon sheath infection

It is important that diagnosis of this condition is made correctly as urgent washout is required to prevent long-term damage to the flexor tendons within the sheath.

The main symptom is pain, with associated swelling and loss of movement in the affected finger.

Kanavel's four cardinal signs help to make the diagnosis:[14]

1. Fusiform sausage-like swelling.
2. Finger held in flexed position.
3. Pain on trying to extend the flexed finger passively.
4. Percussion tenderness along the course of the flexor tendon.

Ligament problems
Gamekeeper's thumb/skier's thumb

This is an ulnar collateral ligament (UCL) injury of the thumb MCP joint. Gamekeeper's thumb probably describes a more chronic attrition injury to the collateral ligament as a result of repetitive actions.[15] Skier's thumb demonstrates clearly how an abduction injury to the thumb MCP joint can lead to an acute tear or avulsion of the UCL.

An acute injury will present with a painful, swollen and bruised thumb localizing to the MCP joint. In a chronic injury the swelling and bruising would have disappeared and the pain may then only occur with heavier activities. Patients will note a reduced grip strength.

The findings at inspection will therefore be determined by the age of the injury. In an older injury there may be no bruising, but swelling may persist. The thumb may lie in a slightly abducted position at the MCP joint.

Palpation will often demonstrate tenderness at the origin, path and insertion of the UCL on the ulnar side

(a)

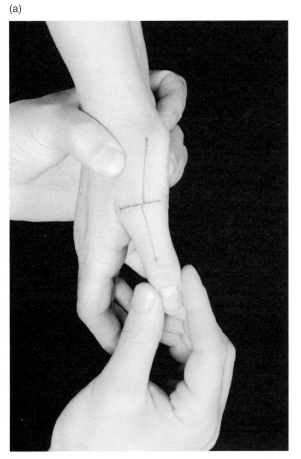

(b)

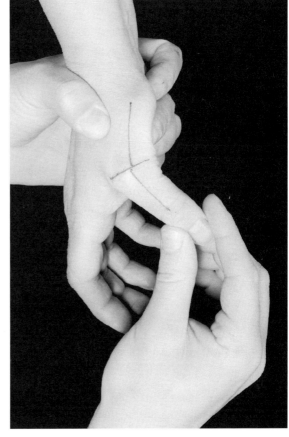

Figure 5.25 a and **b** Stressing the MCP joint to reveal a UCL rupture.

of the joint. Examining range of movement may not demonstrate any problems with flexion or extension of the MCP joint. However, specific attention must be paid to the abnormal movement of instability that may result from a damaged UCL. The thumb is stressed in a radial direction. This is carried out with the joint slightly flexed (10–15°) to 'unlock it', as, even with a torn UCL, the joint may be stable in full extension. With radial deviation the MCP joint will open up; a comparison with the normal side will highlight this more clearly. A firm endpoint should be sought.

A longitudinal line may be drawn along the metacarpal, continuing along the proximal phalanx. A transverse line perpendicular to this on the dorsum of the MCP joint may also be drawn. On stressing the joint these lines may make more obvious to the clinician how much angular deformation occurs (Figure 5.25).

In an acute setting the joint will be too painful to carry out this test. The options are then to let the injury and its discomfort settle down before reassessing or, if a definite injury is suspected and there is no radiological corroboration, local anaesthetic may be infiltrated to create a block before stressing the joint.

The same process may be carried out to assess the potential for other ligamentous injuries affecting the joints of the hand, whether radial collateral or ulnar collateral injuries of MCP, PIP or DIP joints.

Evaluation of vascular supply

Vascular integrity of the hand can be assessed using Allen's test. This can be performed on the whole hand or on individual digits. An example of where it is important to test the whole hand is with excision of a volar ganglion or a surgical approach to the scaphoid tubercle where there is a chance of damaging the radial artery. In this case the presence of a good ulnar artery supply to the hand should be established before embarking on surgery. In cases of revision surgery for Dupuytren's disease, a digital Allen's test should be performed.

The **Allen's test** is performed with the patient's elbow flexed and the forearm supinated. Next, the ulnar and radial arteries are palpated with the thumbs of the examiner's hands. Ask the patient to open and close the fists a few times before keeping them clenched. This action exsanguinates the blood from the hand. The radial and ulnar arteries are then simultaneously compressed by the examiner's thumbs. The patient is then instructed to open the hand. It should appear blanched because the arterial supply is occluded. Next, release compression from one of the arteries and observe the colour to the hand. If the released artery is contributing significantly to perfusion, the normal colour should return to the palm and fingers within a few seconds. If it does not then it is likely that perfusion via that artery is reduced. The test is repeated, this time releasing the other artery. In 75% of patients the ulnar artery predominates over the radial artery. However, either artery should be able to perfuse the hand on its own in the majority of patients.

The **digital Allen's test** is performed in a similar manner, but this time the digital arteries are occluded on either side of the finger being tested.

Summary

Summary of clinical examination of the hand
Step 1
Perform the screen test
Step 2
Subsequent path of examination is based on findings on screening, e.g. Dupuytren's, rheumatoid, lumps and bumps, nerve lesions

- There are so many varied pathologies in the hand and each necessitates a different pattern of examination
- The easiest way to approach clinical examination of the hand is to have a screen test

that will help to determine the pathology and then tailor the subsequent examination based on the observed findings. For example, a nerve lesion would be examined differently to a patient with Dupuytren's disease or a swelling in the hand.

The **screen test** for picking up hand pathology is as follows.

1. Expose the patient adequately, up to their shoulders, and ask him or her to make a fist and open the hands with palms facing upwards.
2. Make a fist and open the fingers with palms facing downwards.
3. Ask the patient to lift his or her hand over the shoulders, exposing the forearms, and look at the profile and for scars, including around the elbow and axilla.

It is also important to be able to **assess the functions of the hand**, as many surgical decisions are based on function, such as in rheumatoid arthritis.

- 45% grasp, 45% pinch, 5% hook and 5% paperweight.

Types of pinch:

- chuck pinch ('pick this coin up from my hand')
- end or pen pinch ('hold this pen')
- side or key pinch ('hold this key').

Then, for grasp, ask the patient to 'shake my hand and grasp tight'.

Tips for assessing patients with a swelling in the hand

The diagnosis of a swelling in the hand depends to a large degree on the location of the swelling.

Volar

Lumps on the volar side of the hand are inclusion dermoid cysts, ganglion of A1 pulley and giant cell tumour of the flexor sheath usually located in relation to the proximal phalanx.

A swelling in relation to the radial artery may be the volar ganglion which comes from the STT joint. If considering surgery, remember to perform Allen's test to check for perfusion from the radial and ulnar arteries.

Dorsal

On the dorsum of the hand possible swellings are:

- Dorsal ganglion over the wrist
- Rheumatoid nodules on the extensor surface
- Gouty tophi
- Subungual exostosis under the nail
- Heberden's nodes over DIP joint
- Mucous cyst in relation to the DIP joint
- Bouchard's nodes in relation to the PIP joint
- Carpometacarpal boss.

Tips on examining patients with Dupuytren's disease

When assessing a patient with Dupuytren's disease the important points to obtain are as follows.

a. Signs of aggressive disease:

  - Early age of onset
  - Garrod's pads
  - Involvement of other sites such as feet, penis and other hand
  - Radial involvement.

b. Indications for surgery:

  - Positive table top test
  - MCP joint flexion contracture ($>30°$)
  - PIP joint flexion contracture.

Examination of Dupuytren's disease

Step 1
Palpate the cords and rest of the palm

Step 2
Look for Garrod's pads

Step 3
Perform table top test (failure to put hand flat on table indicates either a PIP joint flexion contracture or an MCP joint flexion contracture)

Step 4
Measure fixed flexion deformities at MCP joint and the PIP joint using a goniometer

Step 5
Ask the patient about family history, age of onset and if any other parts of the body are affected

---

Remember, when examining a patient who has had previous surgery it is important to perform Allen's test on the digits to assess for neurovascular damage.

Tips for examining the rheumatoid hand

It is important to know all the possible abnormalities that can occur in rheumatoid disease affecting the hand. With this knowledge description becomes easier.

Examination of the rheumatoid hand

Step 1
Ask the patient to lift arms, if possible above the head, to gain a general impression of shoulder and elbow function and also to look for rheumatoid nodules

Step 2
Work from proximal to distal, first on the extensor side and then proximal to distal on the flexor side, stating all the abnormalities

Step 3
Perform functional tests of the hand

On the extensor side from proximal to distal the possible abnormalities are:

- Rheumatoid nodules
- DRUJ instability with caput ulnae (piano key sign)
- Extensor tendon rupture (Vaughan-Jackson syndrome)
- MCP joint subluxation and ulnar deviation
- Finger deformities such as mallet finger, Boutonnière's deformity, swan neck deformity and Z-deformity of the thumb.

On the flexor side abnormalities are:

- Thickening of the carpal tunnel resulting in carpal tunnel syndrome
- Thenar wasting
- Tendon ruptures such as FPL (Mannerfelt lesion)
- Trigger finger.

Acknowledgement

I would like to acknowledge the help of Mr Michael Gale in the preparation of this chapter.

References

1   Hueston JT. The table top test. *Hand* 1982;**14**:100–103.

2   Elson RA. Rupture of the central slip of the extensor hood of the finger. A test for early diagnosis. *J Bone Joint Surg (Br)* 1986; **68B**:229–231.

3   Bunnell S. Ischaemic contracture, local, in the hand. *J Bone Joint Surg (Am)* 1953;**35A**:88–101.

4   Brewerton DA. Hand deformities in rheumatoid disease. *Ann Rheum Dis* 1957;**16**:183–197.

5   Zancolli E. *Structural and Dynamic Bases of Hand Surgery*, 2nd edition. Philadelphia: Lippincott, 1979.

6   Welsh RP, Hastings DE. Swan neck deformity in rheumatoid arthritis of the hand. *Hand* 1977;**9**:109–116.

7   Nalebuff EA. Diagnosis, classification and management of rheumatoid thumb deformities. *Bull Hosp Joint Dis* 1968;**29**:119–137.

8   Mannerfelt L, Norman O. Attrition ruptures of flexor tendons in rheumatoid arthritis caused by bony spurs in the carpal tunnel. A clinical and radiological study. *J Bone Joint Surg (Br)* 1969;**51**: 270–277.

9   Vaughan-Jackson OJ. Rupture of extensor tendons by attrition at the inferior radio-ulnar joint. *J Bone Joint Surg (Br)* 1948;**30B**:528.

10 Roberts ME, Wright V, Hill AG, Mehra AC. Psoriatic arthritis: follow-up study. *Ann Rheum Dis* 1976; **35**:206–212.

11 Mensch A. Spatruptur der sehne des extensor pollicis longus. *Munch Med Wochenschr* 1925;**72**:836.

12 Magnussen PA, Harvey FJ, Tonkin MA. Extensor indicis proprius transfer for rupture of the extensor pollicis longus tendon. *J Bone Joint Surg (Br)* 1990;**72B**:881–883.

13 Quinnell RC. Conservative management of trigger finger. *Practitioner* 1980;**224**:187–190.

14 Kanavel AB. *Infections of the Hand*, 7th edition. London: Baillière, Tindall & Cox, 1939.

15 Campbell CS. Gamekeeper's thumb. *J Bone Joint Surg (Br)* 1955;**37B**:148–149.

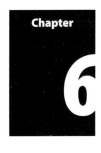

Chapter

6

Examination of the peripheral nerves in the hand and upper limb

John E. D. Wright and L. Chris Bainbridge

Introduction

Productive examination of the peripheral nerves in the upper limb is based on a comprehensive knowledge of the anatomy of the brachial plexus and the course of the nerves as they pass distally. Examination of the terminal components of the nerves informs us of the proximal pathology. Knowledge of dermatomal and specific sensory nerve cutaneous supply is essential (Figure 6.1).

Examination is guided by a full history. Hand dominance, main occupation, hobbies and past injuries or neurological disorders should be documented, as well as the patient's age. Age significantly affects both the quality and quantity of nerve recovery following injury. It is better in children and young adults; the rate of nerve regeneration in children is 2–3 mm per day, compared with 1–2 mm in adults.

The nature of the injury, e.g. knife or hydraulic press, should be clearly documented, as this will have a profound impact on the results of nerve surgery. In the elective situation, localization of the site of injury along the course of the nerve may be comparatively difficult. However, enquiry should be made about previous injuries or operations in the upper limb. The timing of injury or the evolution and duration of a compressive neuropathy are important. For example, if the duration of carpal tunnel compression symptoms is less than 10 months, there is a significant chance of recovery utilizing conservative measures.[1]

Comorbidities (especially diabetes, thyroid disease and other endocrine disease) should be elicited, as compression syndromes (in particular carpal tunnel syndrome) are commonly associated with systemic disease. Smoking and alcohol intake are other factors to be considered. The pattern and frequency of analgesic usage may forewarn the surgeon about the severity of the problem and provide information on diurnal variation in symptoms.

Specific symptoms of nerve disease

Patients sometimes find it difficult to localize neurological symptoms specifically. Patients may describe pain along the course of a specific nerve, and the distribution of tingling, paraesthesia and numbness can be diagnostic, but there may be significant variation. Symptoms in the radial three digits are strongly suggestive of carpal tunnel compression, but symptoms may be just in the middle finger as these fibres are most superficial in the medial nerve. It is also important to differentiate whether symptoms are in the distribution of a specific nerve or the radicular distribution of a cervical root. Symptoms of nerve compression are often exacerbated at night, and the temporal pattern of symptoms should be elicited.

Difficulty with fine tasks, like buttons or dropping objects, is often described: sensory loss and muscle weakness both contribute to a lack of dexterity. However, pain, particularly in the first carpometacarpal (CMC) joint, needs to be excluded as the underlying cause of poor hand function.

Examination of specific nerves

Compression neuropathy and traumatic injury are the two main causes of peripheral nerve symptoms in the upper limb. Knowing a logical sequence of examination for each of the three main nerves and their branches will enable the examiner to identify the site of pathology in the course of the nerve. With knowledge from the elicited history, examination should follow the following pattern: inspection,

Examination Techniques in Orthopaedics, Second Edition, ed. Nick Harris and Fazal Ali. Published by Cambridge University Press. © Cambridge University Press 2014.

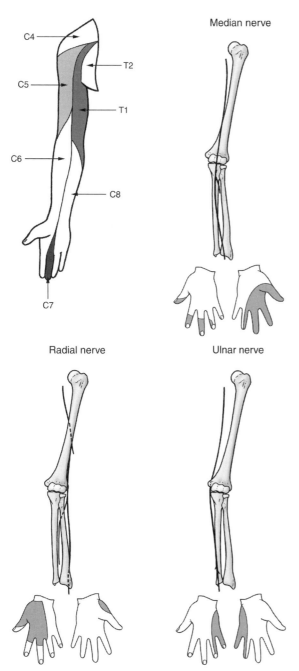

Figure 6.1 Dermatomes of the upper limb and the sensory supply of the median, radial and ulnar nerves. Note the general course of the nerve in the arm.

sensory testing, palpation, motor testing and provocation tests. There are common sites of compression for compressive neuropathies, and the syndromes for each nerve are described below (Table 6.1). The aim of examination for traumatic injuries is to identify which parts of the nerve are injured, which are still functioning and assess for recovery.

Median nerve

The common syndromes associated with compression of the median nerve are pronator syndrome, anterior interosseous nerve (AIN) syndrome and carpal tunnel syndrome. It is important to know the common sites of pathology so that they can be examined specifically. Remember that the site of compression may be in the proximal forearm, but the diagnostic testing is of a function in the hand.

Potential sites of injury/compression

Pronator syndrome

Sites of proximal median nerve compression from proximal to distal are as follows.

- **Ligament of Struthers**: this is an aberrant ligament which, when present, lies between the medial epicondyle of the humerus and a bony spur located 5 cm proximally on the humeral shaft. The median nerve, along with the brachial artery and vein, runs between the ligament and the humerus, where it is liable to compression (Figure 6.2).
- **Lacertus fibrosus**: along its course from the elbow into the forearm, the median nerve runs beneath the thick lacertus fibrosus (extending from biceps tendon to the forearm fascia).
- **Pronator teres (PT)**: between the superficial and deep heads.
- Fibrous arch of the **flexor digitorum superficialis** (FDS) muscle.

Any one or any combination of these are possible sources of compression.

Carpal tunnel syndrome

The site of compression of carpal tunnel syndrome is within the carpal tunnel beneath the transverse carpal ligament.

Examination routine for the median nerve

Inspection: wasting of the thenar muscles, in particular abductor pollicis brevis (APB), is best seen with the hand in profile (Figure 6.3). The scar of a previous carpal tunnel decompression may not be obvious unless specifically sought.

Sensation: the median nerve terminal branch can be tested by sensation at the tip of the index finger.

Table 6.1 Compression syndromes of peripheral nerves in the hand and upper limb

	Median nerve	Radial nerve	Ulnar nerve
Proximal – sensory	Pronator syndrome	Radial tunnel syndrome	Mild cubital tunnel syndrome
Proximal – motor	Anterior interosseous nerve syndrome	Posterior interosseous nerve syndrome	Severe cubital tunnel syndrome
Distal	Carpal tunnel syndrome	Wartenberg's syndrome	Guyon's canal compression

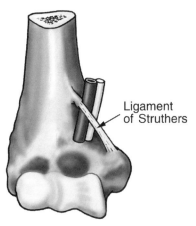

Ligament of Struthers

Figure 6.2 The ligament of Struthers and its relationship to the median nerve and the brachial artery.

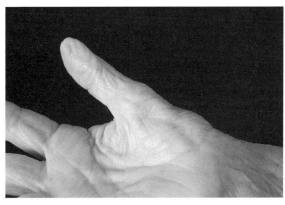

Figure 6.3 Gross wasting of the thenar muscles in a patient with median nerve palsy.

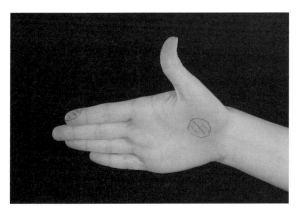

Figure 6.4 The two areas to test for median nerve sensation. In low lesions the sensation in the base of the thenar eminence is preserved.

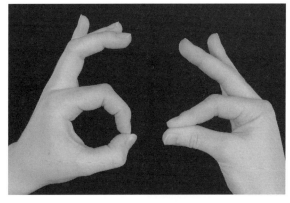

Figure 6.5 The OK sign. Note that in the presence of an anterior interosseous nerve palsy the FDP to the index finger and the FPL is affected, and therefore the patient is unable to make a complete 'O'.

The presence or absence of sensation over the base of the thenar eminence will differentiate between proximal compression and compression within the carpal tunnel. The palmar cutaneous branch of the median nerve arises about 3–5 cm proximal to the wrist crease and runs above the level of the transverse carpal ligament. Consequently, in classical carpal tunnel syndrome, normal sensation is expected in the skin over the thenar eminence. Numbness at this site indicates a more proximal level of nerve compression (Figure 6.4). There are no cutaneous sensory fibres in the AIN.

Palpation: rarely, tenderness over the median nerve in the proximal forearm can be elicited at one of the anatomical sites of compression described above.

Table 6.2 Median nerve motor testing

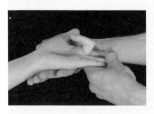

FDS – place hand in palm or on table, hold fingers in extension except middle finger and ask the patient to bend the finger. Active flexion at the PIP joint demonstrates FDS function

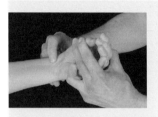

FCR – ask patient to flex wrist against resistance; observe, and palpate tension in the FCR tendon

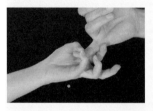

OP – ask the patient to touch tip of thumb to little finger and ask them to resist you pulling fingers apart

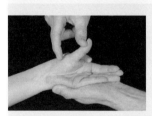

APB – cradle the patient's hand in yours or place it on the table. Ask the patient to raise/abduct the thumb towards the ceiling and maintain it against resistance. Feel the APB, which is the most radial of the thenar muscles

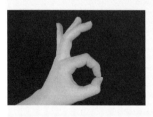

OK sign – ask the patient to make a circle with the thumb and index finger and pinch the tips together. If the AIN-innervated FPL and FDP are deficient, the patient extends at the interphalangeal joints and pinches with the thumb and finger pulps

APB, abductor pollicis brevis; AIN, anterior interosseous nerve; FCR, flexor carpi radialis; FDP, flexor digitorum profundus; FDS, flexor digitorum superficialis; FPL, flexor pollicis longus; OP, opponens pollicis; PIP, proximal interphalangeal.

Motor testing (Table 6.2): a logical sequence of testing is to examine the more proximally innervated muscles first and then test the muscles supplied by the AIN. Flexor carpi radialis (FCR) and FDS are supplied by the median nerve in the forearm, proximal to the carpal tunnel. APB and opponens pollicis (OP) are supplied by the median nerve distal to the carpal tunnel. Testing these four muscles in sequence will identify the level of pathology. The classic test for the AIN is the OK sign or Kiloh–Nevin sign.[2] The patient is asked to make a circle with the thumb and index finger and pinch the tips together; if the AIN-innervated flexor pollicis longus (FPL) and flexor digitorum profundus (FDP) are deficient, the patient extends at the interphalangeal (IP) joints and pinches with the thumb and finger pulps (Figure 6.5).

Provocative tests: it is good practice to perform these at the end of the examination as they can cause discomfort to the patient. The sites of specific compression syndromes and provocation tests for them are outlined below.

Provocation tests for pronator syndrome

1. The patient's elbow is flexed and the forearm pronated. The patient is then instructed to supinate the forearm forcibly, against resistance. The biceps tendon and lacertus fibrosus become taut and may exacerbate the symptoms.
2. The patient's forearm is placed in full supination and the patient is instructed to pronate the arm forcibly against resistance. This will tighten PT and increase any median nerve entrapment.
3. Forceful flexion of the proximal interphalangeal (PIP) joint of the middle finger against resistance will similarly increase any compression against the arch of the FDS.

Provocation tests for carpal tunnel syndrome

1. Phalen's test – placing the patient's wrists in a maximally flexed position reproduces the patient's symptoms. This is a time-dependent test, so the shorter time it takes for the patient to notice symptoms the more sensitive the test.
2. Reverse Phalen's – with the wrist maximally extended, the symptoms are reproduced.
3. Paley and McMurtry described a method where direct pressure applied over the median nerve at the level of the distal wrist crease reproduced the symptoms within 30 seconds to 2 minutes.[3]

There is no wrist movement involved in this test. Therefore it is a useful provocation test to employ among patients with painful wrist conditions or wrist stiffness. Durkan described a modification of this, advising that pressure should be applied using both thumbs over the carpal tunnel itself.[4]

4. Other less common tests include the tourniquet test and straight arm raising (SAR) test.[5] In these, the symptoms of nerve compression may be precipitated by increasing the nerve ischaemia by either applying a tourniquet or simply elevating the arm above the head level with wrist in neutral position.

5. Tinel's test – percussion over the median nerve reproduces symptoms. The best place to percuss the nerve is just proximal to the wrist crease at the point at which the nerve enters the carpal tunnel.

Radial nerve

The radial nerve can be injured by trauma or compression. Classical sites of injury are either above the elbow (in the axilla or the spiral groove of the humerus), or below the elbow in the forearm. Trauma – blunt, penetrating or iatrogenic – can injure the radial nerve as it passes around the humerus. The common compression syndromes are posterior interosseous nerve (PIN) syndrome, radial tunnel syndrome and Wartenberg's syndrome.[6] Following the examination sequence of inspection, palpation, sensory testing, motor testing and provocative tests, will enable the examiner to identify the level of radial nerve pathology.

Potential sites of injury/compression

Above the elbow

Common causes of radial nerve injury are a spiral fracture of the distal humerus (Holstein–Lewis injury), iatrogenic injury at the time of surgery for stabilization of a humeral fracture and external pressure (including tourniquet injury). The examiner should be alerted to possible radial nerve pathology by scars in the upper arm, either from trauma or surgery. A high injury of the radial nerve before it divides will affect both the superficial sensory branch and the PIN.

Around the elbow

The two classic radial nerve compression syndromes described are radial tunnel syndrome and PIN syndrome. These are sometimes difficult syndromes to diagnose and their exact aetiology and management are unclear. The major difference between the syndromes is the presence of pain and motor weakness in the PIN-innervated muscles with PIN syndrome, and the presence of pain but without weakness in radial tunnel syndrome.

The motor branch of the radial nerve divides above the supinator muscle and the PIN passes through the two heads of the supinator in the so-called 'radial tunnel'. The proximal boundary of the supinator is thickened and termed the arcade of Frohse. Other anatomic structures that can compress the radial nerve are believed to be fibrous bands in front of the radiocapitellar joint, a leash of vessels from the anterior recurrent radial artery and the fibrous proximal edge of extensor carpi radialis brevis (ECRB).

The main differential diagnosis for these syndromes is lateral epicondylitis. In both diagnoses the patient may report pain in the lateral aspect of the elbow, radiating to the forearm. Classically, the point tenderness for lateral epicondylitis (the insertion of ECRB just anterior to the lateral epicondyle) is more proximal and posterior than the tenderness of palpating the radial tunnel.

It is important when examining for compression or injury to the PIN to assess for radial deviation on extension of the wrist. The reason for this is that extensor carpi radialis longus (ECRL) is supplied by the radial nerve and ECRB by the PIN, before it enters the radial tunnel; however, extensor carpi ulnaris (ECU) is supplied by the PIN after entry to the radial tunnel. Therefore, complete weakness of wrist extension suggests a very high radial nerve injury, while weakness of ulnar deviation and wrist extension, but good power of radial deviation and wrist extension, suggests that the level of compression or injury is between the innervation of ECRL and ECU.

Around the wrist

The terminal sensory branch of the radial nerve (radial superficial sensory nerve) passes under brachioradialis to emerge through the deep fascia in the distal forearm to supply sensation over the dorsum of the first web space.

The nerve is vulnerable when an anterior Henry approach is used to plate a radial fracture and the scar for this should alert the examiner to possible sensory disturbance in the distribution of the nerve. The nerve can also be compressed as it passes over the radius at the level of the wrist. Trauma at this level, with associated pain or paraesthesia over the dorsum of the first web space, was first described by Wartenberg in 1930.[7] The patient may report a history of wearing a new watch or having been handcuffed, as both can cause irritation of the superficial radial sensory nerve.

Examination routine for the radial nerve

Inspection: observe the posture of the wrist and identify any potentially relevant scars. Inspection may reveal a 'dropped wrist' posture and possibly the use of a wrist extension splint.

Sensation: testing for sensation in the first web space in the dorsum of the hand will identify whether there is pathology either in the main radial nerve trunk or in the superficial sensory branch (Figure 6.6). There are no cutaneous sensory fibres in the PIN, so, if there is weakness of PIN-innervated muscles but normal sensation in the superficial sensory branch distribution, the pathology is distal to the bifurcation of the nerve in the PIN.

Palpation: if lateral epicondylitis or compression in the radial tunnel is suspected then palpation for tenderness on the lateral side of the elbow will be helpful in differentiating between them. Distally, examination may reveal tenderness along the course of the superficial sensory nerve with a positive Tinel's test. This must be differentiated from the tenderness of De Quervain's disease, which is slightly more distal.

Motor testing (Table 6.3): the radial nerve supplies the wrist extensors and extensors of the metacarpophalangeal (MCP) joints of the fingers (Figure 6.7). It is logical to examine the muscles in the order in which they are innervated. The most proximal muscle to be tested is brachioradialis, which is visualized and palpated by asking the patient to flex the elbow against resistance when held at 90°. Then the muscles ECRL and ECU are tested as described above to identify whether the pathology is above or below the bifurcation of the radial nerve. The more distally innervated muscles of the PIN are the extensor pollicis longus (EPL) and extensor indicis (EI), which can be tested by demonstrating retropulsion of the thumb or index finger pointing.

A common error is to believe incorrectly that the patient can fully extend their fingers, when the extension is only at the IP joints, but not the MCP joints. IP joint extension is a function of the median and ulnar nerves.

Provocative tests: finally, if compression within the radial tunnel is considered, provocation is

Table 6.3 Radial nerve motor testing

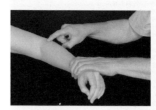

Brachioradialis – is visualized and palpated by asking the patient to flex the elbow against resistance when held at 90°

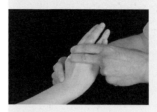

ECRL – the patient is asked to extend and radially deviate their wrist against resistance

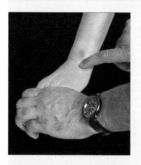

ECU – the patient is asked to extend and ulnarly deviate the wrist against resistance

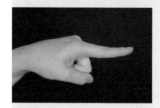

EI – the patient is asked to flex the ulnar three fingers and point with the index finger

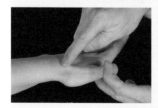

EPL – the patient is asked to place the hand palm down on the table and then lift the thumb, called retropulsion of the thumb. Palpate the EPL

ECRL, extensor carpi radialis longus; ECU, extensor carpi ulnaris; EI, extensor indicis; EPL, extensor pollicis longus.

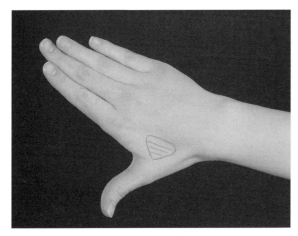

Figure 6.6 Area to test for radial nerve sensation.

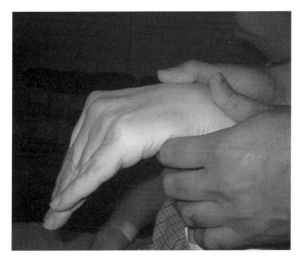

Figure 6.7 Inability to extend the fingers at the MCP joints in patient with radial nerve palsy.

performed. Resisted active supination with the elbow in extension will increase the pressure beneath the arcade of Frohse. This will increase the pain if the PIN is already being compressed. A positive test is indicated by reproduction of pain in the proximal forearm.

Ulnar nerve

The ulnar nerve may be injured by trauma or primary neurological disease, but the most common cause for dysfunction is compression either in the cubital tunnel behind the medial epicondyle or compression in Guyon's canal at the wrist.

Classically, examination is aiming to identify whether there is a 'high' or 'low' lesion of the ulnar

nerve. In a high, or proximal lesion, the extrinsic and intrinsic muscles are affected. In a low, or distal lesion, only the intrinsic muscles are involved. Detailed knowledge of the anatomy and a structured examination can identify the level of pathology along the course of the nerve.

Potential sites of injury/compression
Around the elbow

Compression around the elbow can be caused by the following structures:

- **The arcade of Struthers**: a fascial band extending from the medial intermuscular septum to the medial head of triceps.
- The **medial intermuscular septum** itself.
- Exostoses or osteophytes of the **medial epicondyle**.
- The **cubital tunnel and Osbourne's ligament**: a fascial band bridging the two heads of flexor carpi ulnaris (FCU) muscle.
- **Anconeus epitrochlearis**: an accessory muscle.

At the wrist

Compression at the wrist is in Guyon's canal. Here the ulnar nerve passes between the transverse carpal ligament and the volar carpal ligament before passing around the hook of hamate.

Examination routine for the ulnar nerve

Inspection: the appearance of a hand with severe ulnar nerve pathology is usually easy to identify from the combination of muscle wasting and finger posture. Recently, the rectangle palm sign has been described, showing that the normal square palm shape becomes rectangular with severe wasting of the hypothenar eminence and first dorsal interosseous muscle.[8] Proximal dysfunction can cause wasting of the volar ulnar side of the forearm – FCU and FDP. Sometimes the wasting of the interossei (guttering), the hypothenar eminence and the first dorsal interosseous can be subtle (Figure 6.8). Screening with the shoulders and elbows flexed 90° may reveal the wasting of the hypothenar eminence. However, further inspection with elevation of the elbows is required to fully inspect the posterior aspect of the elbow for the scars of cubital tunnel decompression (Figure 6.9).

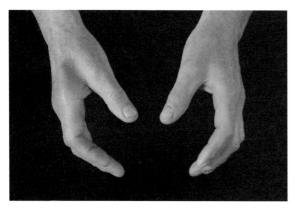

Figure 6.8 Ulnar nerve palsy resulting in gross wasting of the first dorsal interosseous muscle of this patient's right hand.

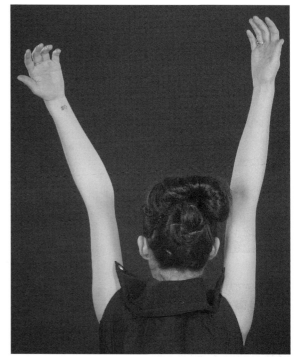

Figure 6.9 When inspecting it is useful to ask the patient to lift the arms so that the elbows can be inspected for scars. In this case this patient also demonstrates a significant cubitus valgus.

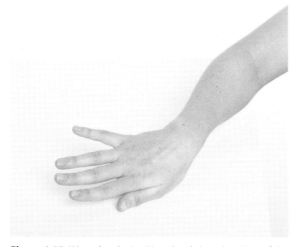

Figure 6.10 Wartenberg's sign. Note the abducted position of the little finger due to weakness of the third palmar interosseous muscle. The EDM pulls the finger into an extended position.

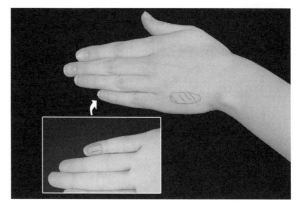

Figure 6.11 Areas to test for ulnar nerve sensation. In low lesions the sensation on the dorsal surface of the fifth metacarpal is preserved.

Wartenberg's sign (1930) is considered one of the earliest signs. In this the little finger adopts an abducted posture – due to weakness of the third palmar interosseous muscle, and its function being overpowered by the extensor digiti minimi (EDM), which is PIN-innervated (Figure 6.10). 'Clawing' of the fingers or 'benediction hand' (Duchenne's sign, which was first described in 1867) is a classic feature of ulnar nerve dysfunction. It is important to identify hyperextension at the MCP joint in association with flexion at the PIP joint – the opposite of lumbrical function. The index and middle fingers are less affected, as the median nerve innervates the first two lumbricals. Unlike any other peripheral nerve lesions, the claw deformity is exaggerated with more distal ulnar nerve lesions, as FDP to the little and ring

Table 6.4 Ulnar nerve motor testing

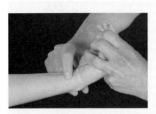

FCU – the patient is asked to flex the wrist against resistance; the tension in the tendon of FCU can be seen and palpated

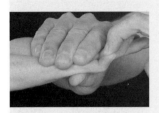

FDP – stabilizes the patient's little finger PIP joint in extension; feel for active flexion of the DIP joint against resistance

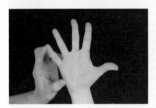

ADM – ask the patient to hold the hands palms facing their face and spread open their finger. Push the little finger towards the ring finger. Weakness results in the inability of the little finger to maintain its position

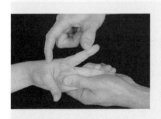

First dorsal interosseous – hold the patient's hand with the index finger uppermost. Ask them to lift the finger (abduct) then resist your pressure as you span the finger with your other hand as you palpate the muscle belly

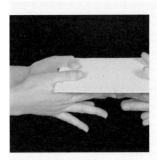

Froment's test – the patient is asked to grasp a piece of paper in the first web space, between their extended thumb and extended fingers. Normally the first dorsal interosseous and adductor pollicis would be able to resist the examiner pulling the paper out and the thumb remains extended. However, if the ulnar nerve is deficient, the patient will recruit the AIN-innervated FPL to grasp the paper and the thumb IP joint will flex

ADM, abductor digiti minimi; AIN, anterior interosseous nerve; FCU, flexor carpi ulnaris; FDP, flexor digitorum profundus; FPL, flexor pollicis longus.

fingers (which are partly responsible for the clawing) are innervated in the proximal forearm. This is called the 'ulnar paradox'. The paradox also manifests after a high ulnar nerve injury. In this instance, the claw deformity initially worsens as the nerve recovers and starts to reinnervate the FDP.

Sensation: sensory testing can differentiate between a 'high' and a 'low' ulnar nerve lesion. The ulnar nerve gives off a sensory branch 5 cm proximal to the wrist, whose cutaneous territory is over the dorsum of the fifth metacarpal (Figure 6.11). If sensation is altered here it suggests that the pathology is more proximal, usually at the cubital tunnel. In this case, sensation at the tip of the

little finger is also altered. If sensation is intact over the dorsum of the fifth metacarpal, but altered in the tip of the little finger, the pathology is most likely to be in Guyon's canal (a low lesion).

Palpation: tenderness may be elicited over either the cubital tunnel or Guyon's canal. The former should be differentiated from medial epicondylitis, which can coexist.

Motor testing (Table 6.4): the only muscles supplied by the ulnar nerve in the forearm are FCU and FDP to the little and ring fingers. These will be intact with a low lesion and can be tested by resisted wrist flexion, palpating the tendon of FCU, followed by resisted flexion of the distal interphalangeal (DIP) joint of the little finger. Inability to flex the DIP joint of the little and ring finger was described by Pollock in 1919. The same information can be gained by asking a patient to make a fist and observe whether they are able to tuck the little finger into the palm.

There are numerous ways of testing the intrinsic muscles of the hand innervated by the ulnar nerve. Simply crossing the fingers is an easy test and very useful in children. Alternatively, asking the patient to press their abducted little fingers together can easily demonstrate unilateral weakness of the hypothenar eminence. Rarely, only the deep branch of the ulnar nerve is

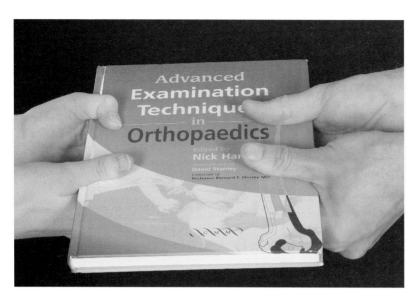

Figure 6.12 Froment's test. The patient is asked to grasp a piece of paper or thin book between extended finger and thumb. Because adductor pollicis (ulnar nerve) is not working FPL is recruited to perform the task.

compromised and in this situation the hypothenar muscles are spared but the rest of the intrinsic muscles are affected.

The first dorsal interosseous can be tested for power and the muscle belly palpated by holding the patient's hand, asking them to abduct their index finger; resist the movement with your middle finger and palpate the muscle with your thumb.

Provocative tests: forced flexion of the elbow can increase pressure in the cubital tunnel and cause sensory disturbance in the ulnar nerve distribution. Tinel's test with percussion of the ulnar nerve over the cubital tunnel and over Guyon's canal can be helpful; however, in many 'normal' subjects percussion over the ulnar nerve at the elbow can cause sensory disturbance into the little and ring finger – the funny bone!

The classical test for the ulnar nerve was described by Froment (1915). The patient is asked to grasp a piece of paper in the first web space, between their extended thumb and extended fingers. Normally the first dorsal interosseous and adductor pollicis would be able to resist the examiner pulling the paper out and the thumb remains extended. However, if the ulnar nerve is deficient the patient will recruit the AIN-innervated FPL to grasp the paper and the thumb IP joint will flex (Figure 6.12).

Martin–Gruber anastomosis

Contrary to popular teaching, the innervation pattern in the hand and forearm is not sacrosanct. Crossover of nerve fibres between the three major nerves in the upper limb is possible.

The most common exchange of fibres is between the median and ulnar nerves in the forearm. This is called the Martin–Gruber anastomosis.[9] It is believed to be present in 15–20% of individuals. In this, motor fibres from the median nerve cross over to the ulnar nerve in the proximal forearm. Clinically, this becomes significant, as normal intrinsic muscle function may exist in spite of the ulnar nerve being injured above the level of the anastomosis.

A similar sharing of sensory fibres in the hand can exist between these two nerves. This is due to the Riche–Cannieu anastomosis.

Other peripheral nerves

The other terminal nerves of the brachial plexus that supply the upper limb are the axillary nerve and the musculocutaneous nerve.

Axillary nerve

This nerve supplies the deltoid muscle as well as teres minor and the long head of triceps. To assess this nerve, sensation is tested in the region of the deltoid insertion, the 'regimental patch' area.

Motor function is mainly by testing the deltoid muscle. Passively abduct the shoulder to 90° and then extend it. Ask the patient to resist as you push downward on the arm. Feel the muscle. This tests the posterior deltoid. The central and anterior fibres of the deltoid can be tested by placing the abducted arm in neutral and flexed positions, respectively.

Musculocutaneous nerve

This nerve supplies the biceps brachii, coracobrachialis and the brachialis muscles. Testing the biceps is sufficient to assess the motor function of this nerve. The supinated forearm is placed in 90° of elbow flexion. Further active flexion is resisted by the examiner and the strength of the biceps assessed.

To test supination the forearm is pronated with the elbows flexed to 90° and held firmly at the sides. Active supination is then resisted by the examiner.

The musculocutaneous nerve continues as the lateral cutaneous nerve of the forearm. Therefore sensation can be tested along the lateral aspect of the forearm.

Summary

> **Summary of upper limb peripheral nerve examination**
>
> A quick screen for assessing the peripheral nerves to the hand may be useful, especially in children. Ask the patient to 'point your finger (radial nerve)', 'cross your fingers (ulnar nerve)', 'make an "O" (median nerve)'.

Median nerve

Look	Scars, APB wasting
Feel (sensation)	Tip of index finger; base of thenar eminence
Feel	Proximal forearm over pronator/FDS
Move	FCR FDS APB OP OK sign – AIN
Provocation	Lacertus/PT/FDS – pronator syndrome Tinel's/Phalen's – carpal tunnel syndrome

The sequence allows differentiation between a high median nerve palsy and a low median nerve palsy, such as in carpal tunnel syndrome.

In a high median nerve lesion, both sensory and motor deficit will be present in all the groups. In low median nerve lesions FDS and FCR will be preserved.

With regard to sensory function, in the low lesion the thenar crease area will have preserved sensation as

the palmar branch of the median nerve is superficial to the transverse ligament and is therefore not involved in carpal tunnel syndrome.

In AIN palsy the patient will be unable to perform the OK sign as he or she will be unable to use FPL and FDP to the index finger, both of which are supplied by the AIN.

Radial nerve

Look	Wrist drop, scars, splint
Feel (sensation)	Over dorsum first web space
Feel	Radial tunnel versus lateral epicondyle
Move	Brachioradialis ECRL ECU EI EPL
Provocation	Resisted supination

To differentiate high radial nerve palsy from a PIN palsy – in a high radial nerve injury the power in all these muscles groups will be affected, whereas in a PIN palsy the power in brachioradialis and ECRL will be intact.

Sensation is preserved in a PIN palsy.

Ulnar nerve

Look	FCU wasting, first dorsal interosseous wasting, guttering, hypothenar wasting Claw deformity Wartenberg's sign Rectangle palm Scars
Feel (sensation)	Tip of little finger; dorsum of fifth metacarpal
Feel	Tenderness over cubital tunnel versus medial epicondyle
Move	FCU FDP to little finger ADM First dorsal interosseous Froment's test
Provocation	Tinel's Elbow flexion test

In high ulnar nerve palsy, such as injury around the medial epicondyle, sensation in both areas are affected, whereas in low ulnar nerve problems, such as compression in Guyon's canal, the dorsal branch is preserved, resulting in no loss of sensation in the region of the fifth metacarpal.

In high ulnar nerve lesions the motor power in all muscle groups is affected and Froment's test is positive. In the lower lesion the power in FDP to the little finger and FCU are both preserved.

Differentiation between high and low lesions can also be suspected on inspection. In lower lesions the clawing is much more pronounced than in high ulnar nerve lesions. This is called the ulnar paradox.

References

1   Kaplan SJ, Glickel SZ, Eaton RG. Predictive factors in the non-surgical treatment of carpal tunnel syndrome. *J Hand Surg (Br)* 1990;**15**:106–108.

2   Kiloh LG, Nevin S. Isolated neuritis of the anterior interosseous nerve. *Br Med J* 1952;**1**(4763):850–851.

3   Paley D, McMurtry RY. Median nerve compression test in carpal tunnel syndrome diagnosis reproduces signs and symptoms in affected wrist. *Orthop Rev* 1985;**14**:411.

4   Durkan JA. A new diagnostic test for carpal tunnel syndrome. *J Bone Joint Surg (Am)* 1991; **73**:535–538.

5   Gilliat RW, Wilson TG. A pneumatic-tourniquet test in the carpal-tunnel syndrome. *Lancet* 1953;**265**(6786):595–597.

6   Sarhadi NS, Korday SN, Bainbridge LC. Radial tunnel syndrome: diagnosis and management. *J Hand Surg (Br)* 1998;**23**:617–619.

7   Dellon AL, Mackinnon SE. Radial sensory nerve entrapment in the forearm. *J Hand Surg (Am)* 1986;**11**:199–205.

8   Lloyd N, Sammut D. The rectangular palm sign in ulnar nerve paralysis. *Eur J Plastic Surg* 2012;**35**(7):569–570.

9   Leibovic SJ, Hastings H. Martin–Gruber revisited. *J Hand Surg (Am)* 1992;**17**:47–53.

Further reading

Birch R, Bonney G, Wynn-Parry C B (eds). *Surgical Disorders of the Peripheral Nerves*. Edinburgh: Churchill Livingstone, 1998.

Dawson D, Hallett M, Millender L. *Entrapment Neuropathies*. Boston: Little, Brown, 1990.

Gelberman R (ed). *Operative Nerve Repair and Reconstruction*. Philadelphia: Lippincott, 1991.

The Guarantors of Brain. *Aids to the Examination of the Peripheral Nervous System*. London: Baillière Tindall, 1986.

Wolfe SW, Hotchkiss RN, Pederson WC, Kozin SH. *Green's Operative Hand Surgery*, 6th edition. Amsterdam: Elsevier, 2010.

Examination of the adult spine

Neil Chiverton

History
General history

The majority of adult patients with problems of spinal origin present with complaints of pain in the back and/or legs, with a resultant loss of function.

It is, therefore, as important to understand and record the impact of the perceived pain on the daily work and recreational activities of the patient as it is to enquire about the nature of the pain itself.

One should begin with the patient's occupation, social circumstances (e.g. young children at home, carer for elderly relative, living alone) and sporting activities. Then enquire about the limitations on all of these aspects of daily living with particular reference to days taken off work, time periods of relative immobility and problems coping with household duties. Specific disability scoring systems[1,2] can be used if wished. The patient's age should always be used to help steer thoughts toward a likely diagnosis. Never accept a diagnosis of mechanical back pain in patients outside the age range of 20–55 years without thorough investigation, particularly in the presence of non-mechanical or other atypical symptoms.

With regard to pain, its site, radiation, any precipitating or relieving factors (e.g. posture, cough/sneeze, physical activity), causation, duration and any pain-free intervals should be documented.

It is essential to enquire directly about bowel or bladder dysfunction.

Additionally, it is important to take note of whether the patient considers his/her back problem to be work-related and whether or not there are any legal proceedings pending.

The requirements for analgesics and their effectiveness are a useful guide for the clinician as to the degree of pain experienced by the patient. Also ask about any previous treatments received, such as physiotherapy or chiropractic therapy.

The history-taking should, as always, conclude with a systems review, past medical history, family history, other medications and allergies. With regard to back pain, heredity is also important.

Specific pathologies and their related symptoms
Degenerative disease of the cervical spine

Pain in the neck may be a symptom of cervical spondylosis. Other causes of referred pain to the neck such as shoulder girdle pathology and cervical soft tissue tumours should be considered. Neck stiffness is often reported.

In severe cases of spondylosis patients can present with symptoms of compressive cervical myelopathy, cervical radiculopathy or a mixture of both.

Unsteadiness of gait, limb weakness and sensory disturbance in the upper or lower limbs and urinary dysfunction are the cardinal symptoms of a cervical myelopathy. Patients will commonly report an episodic rather than a gradual deterioration. A thorough history will be required if metabolic, rheumatological and primary neural degenerative disorders are not to be overlooked as potential causes of these symptoms.

Acute cervical disc protrusion can cause myelopathic symptoms, but classically will present with neck and arm pain (brachalgia), the latter resulting from nerve root compression and being the most troublesome to the patient. It is usually described as a burning/toothache type pain. Sensory disturbance is frequently associated. The site of the upper limb pain varies according to the disc level involved – the most

Examination Techniques in Orthopaedics, Second Edition, ed. Nick Harris and Fazal Ali. Published by Cambridge University Press. © Cambridge University Press 2014.

common are the C5/6 and C6/7 disc levels affecting the C6 and C7 nerve roots, respectively. This gives rise to pain and paraesthesiae along the radial aspect of the forearm and into the radial digits. A differential diagnosis based on these symptoms will include peripheral nerve entrapment syndromes, thoracic outlet syndrome, tumours abutting the brachial plexus, idiopathic brachial neuritis and spinal tumours.

A painless but progressive flexion deformity of the cervical spine progressing from a limitation of the forward field of view to difficulty with jaw opening characterizes the cervical spinal manifestations of ankylosing spondylitis.

Degenerative disease of the lumbar spine

A history of low back pain proportional to activity level with periods of exacerbation lasting 2–6 weeks and with radiation into the gluteal and thigh regions only is indicative of so-called 'discogenic pain' from degenerative lower lumbar motion segments. Any associated pain or sensory disturbance in the lower leg or foot suggests the coexistence of a compressive radiculopathy. If the cause of this is an acute intervertebral disc protrusion, the leg pain tends to be severe, unilateral and exacerbated by posture.

The most likely disc level involved can usually be appreciated by ascertaining where the patient reports the symptoms of leg pain, tingling or numbness.

Any reported bowel or bladder disturbance necessitates further investigation, as does reduced perineal sensation.

Neurogenic bladder dysfunction presents as painless overflow incontinence. Symptoms of prostatic hypertrophy in men and stress or urge incontinence in women are not consistent with a cauda equina syndrome, and careful differentiation is essential before urgent investigations are requested unnecessarily.

Back pain with leg pain after a certain period of time walking or standing is suggestive of spinal claudication. Leg symptoms are commonly bilateral and the reported distribution is less specific than with an isolated nerve root compression. Patients with spinal claudication will frequently report improvement in symptoms when walking by leaning on a walking stick, shopping trolley or when walking uphill as these flexed postures increase spinal canal diameter. Complete relief is achieved by sitting for several minutes. In more severe cases rest and night symptoms are present ('restless legs') and neurogenic bladder dysfunction can occur. The differential diagnosis of vascular claudication can be difficult to exclude on history alone but this condition is usually relieved by standing still as well as sitting, and symptoms resolve more rapidly.

Other differential diagnoses include diabetic or alcoholic peripheral neuropathy and spinal tumours.

A combination of radicular and stenotic symptoms as outlined above should raise the possibility of degenerative lumbar spondylolisthesis in which both spinal canal compromise and nerve root entrapment result from the forward slip of one complete vertebra on another.

Degenerative disease of the thoracic spine

Pathology involving the thoracic spine is rare with, for instance, only 0.5% of all disc protrusions occurring in this region. However, they should be considered in anyone complaining of interscapular back pain. The pain has the same nature and precipitating factors as are found in equivalent conditions of the lumbar spine. Radicular symptoms are felt around the chest wall in the distribution of the corresponding intercostal nerve. Myelopathy may affect bladder and bowel function as well as all lower limb muscle groups.

Differential diagnoses include herpes zoster, mediastinal or abdominal pathology and, as always, spinal tumours.

General examination
Inspection

Examination of any localized spinal disorder requires inspection of the entire spine. All patients must undress to their underwear for this to be possible (Figure 7.1).

The usual format for inspection should be followed, first noting any obvious swellings or surgical scars. The erect spinal profile must be assessed for any deformity in the coronal or sagittal plane. Scoliosis will be the result of either a previous developmental deformity or degenerative disease of later onset, or both. A 'forward bend test' may reveal the presence of a rib hump seen commonly in the former, but uncommonly in the latter. Kyphosis in the region of the cervicothoracic junction is typically seen with ankylosing spondylitis, whereas in the thoracic region it is likely to represent either previous Scheuermann's disease or multiple osteoporotic wedge fractures. Loss of lordosis in the lumbar spine is commonly seen in association with protective paravertebral muscle spasm secondary to underlying degenerative disease. Hyperlordosis should raise the suspicion of spondylolisthesis. Hyperlordosis may also be the result of the compensation for a fixed flexion deformity in the hip. Prominent buttocks, shortened trunk and flexed hips and knees may be seen with severe slips. A compensatory lumbar hyperlordosis will be found below a primary thoracic kyphotic deformity.

One should follow this assessment with a check for shoulder asymmetry and pelvic tilt. A plumbline can be used to quantify any coronal imbalance if wished.

Palpation

Palpation along the line of the spine over the paravertebral muscles on both sides is very non-specific, but helps to localize the level of the spine involved (Figure 7.2). Often a region of tenderness on deep palpation is found. Very localized points of tenderness on deep muscle palpation are suggestive of fibromyalgia. Occasionally one may encounter marked superficial tenderness, or a non-anatomic distribution of tenderness that may be non-organic in nature,[3] but one must keep an open mind at this stage as the former sign may be elicited in destructive or infective lesions of the spine.

Palpation should be completed with an abdominal examination to identify any masses, especially a distended neurogenic bladder and the obligatory PR examination of sensation, anal tone and prostate.

Movement

All spinal movements are best assessed actively by instructing the patient on the movements required, but some passive movements are useful.

For the cervical spine, movements of flexion, extension, rotation and lateral flexion should be assessed (Figure 7.3). Flexion and extension are mostly affected by spondylosis. A tendency to hold the head on one side with radicular arm pain when

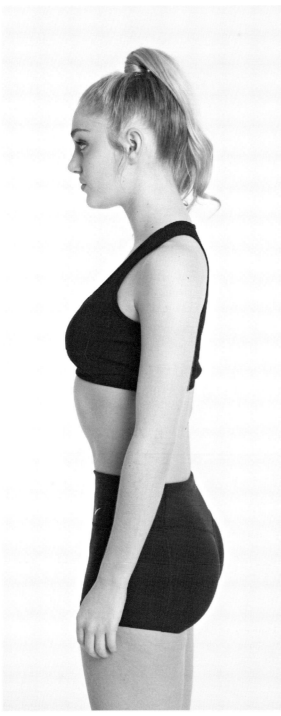

Figure 7.1 Stand patient and inspect the entire spine from the back, sides and front.

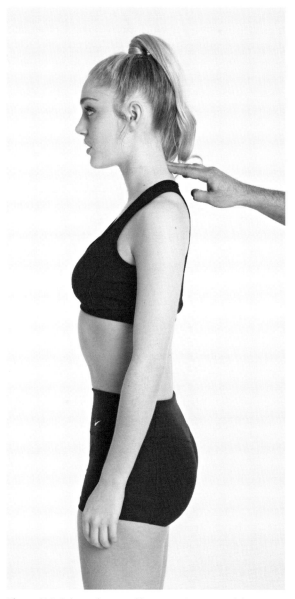

Figure 7.2 Palpate the central bony prominences and the paraspinal areas.

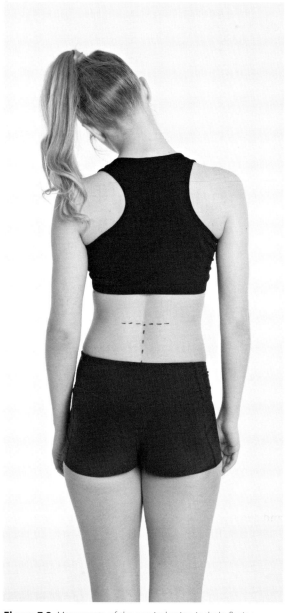

Figure 7.3 Movements of the cervical spine include flexion, extension, rotation and lateral flexion as shown here.

the neck is gently passively laterally flexed to the other side suggests a cervical disc prolapse (on the contralateral side to the active lateral flexion). Normally, only 40% of rotational movement occurs in the subaxial spine so this movement is well preserved in most degenerative disorders.

Facet joint orientation and the splinting effect of the thoracic cage allow for essentially only rotational movement in the thoracic spine. Assessment of this movement is, however, of little diagnostic significance. Conversely, because of the orientation of the facet joints in the lumbar spine, little rotation is possible and flexion/extension movements are examined.

Measurement of forward bending is performed by asking the patient to try and touch their toes. Note and record to what extent they can achieve this (e.g. fingers to knees, mid shin, toes). One should ensure by inspection that the movement is achieved by flexion of the lumbar spine and not the hips only.

Schober's test[4] can be used to provide a more quantitative evaluation of lumbar spine flexion. Mark a horizontal line at the level of the posterior superior iliac spines (PSISs) and a second at a distance of 10 cm above this. On forward flexion this distance should increase by at least 5 cm (Figure 7.4). A modification of this test[5] uses a distal fixed point 5 cm below the PSIS line and the same point above. Limitation of flexion is caused by pain protection or ankylosing spondylitis.

When testing extension stand behind the patient supporting and reassuring him or her. The limitation here can be more marked than limitation of flexion in degenerative disease and is said to indicate facet joint arthrosis.

Lateral flexion can be quantified by recording how far down the legs the tips of the fingers can reach (e.g. to the knee or upper leg, etc.) (Figure 7.5a). Alternatively, the distance from the tip of the fingers to the ground can be measured.

Rotation is performed by fixing the pelvis with the examiner's hands or asking the patient to sit and rotate (Figure 7.5b).

Essential adjuncts to examination of the cervical and lumbar spine are screening movements of the shoulder and hip joints, respectively, to exclude them as a cause of the pain in these regions.

Walk

Before walking the patient it may sometimes be helpful to do a quick screen for the lower lumbar nerve roots by asking patient to squat and get up (assessing quadriceps function, L3), to stand on heels (dorsiflexion of ankles, assessing L4); also ask the patient to stand on one leg and effectively perform Trendelenburg's test (assessing the hip abductors, L5) and, finally, ask him or her to stand on tip toes (assessing plantar flexion of ankle, S1) (Figure 7.6).

Following this, the patient must be observed walking; any neurological gait should be sought (Figure 7.7). An antalgic gait is often noted in the presence of lumbar radiculopathy secondary to disc prolapse. A broad-based unsteady gait can be seen in advanced cervical myelopathy. Sometimes a compensatory scoliosis may be the result of a leg length discrepancy and this may manifest in a short leg gait.

Neurovascular examination

A thorough, orderly examination of sensation (Figure 7.8a), tone, power and reflexes must be performed on all four limbs for problems with the cervical spine and on the lower limbs for thoracolumbar disease. This is most conveniently done with the patient sitting for the cervical spine or lying down for the lumbar spine.

A summary of muscle innervation and reflex values (Table 7.1) and dermatomal distributions (Figure 7.8b) are given.

The MRC booklet on neurological testing[6] or Chapter 1 will give a more detailed description on assessing muscle power. There is a logical sequence to assessing the myotomes of the lower limb (Figure 7.9) and upper limb (Figure 7.10).

Muscle tone can best be assessed by feeling the muscle's resistance to passive stretch. In the upper limb, to do this, support the elbow with one hand and with the other flex and extend the fingers, wrist and elbow in one smooth movement. In the lower limb tone can be assessed by rolling the hip (passively internally and externally rotating it).

When testing reflexes (Figure 7.11a) it is important to remember to examine the **abdominal reflexes** (Figure 7.11b), especially for thoracic spine pathology. This test is performed by stroking the abdomen radially out from the umbilicus in four directions (e.g. 2, 4, 8 and 10 o'clock positions). Normally the underlying muscles will contract involuntarily, resulting in the umbilicus moving in the direction of the quadrant being stroked. Absence of the normal response indicates thoracic spinal compression on the side of the diminished reflex. Remember that the level of the umbilicus is supplied by T10.

All peripheral pulses need to be checked as vascular claudication in the upper or lower limbs can mimic symptoms of radiculopathy or canal stenosis.

(a)

(b)

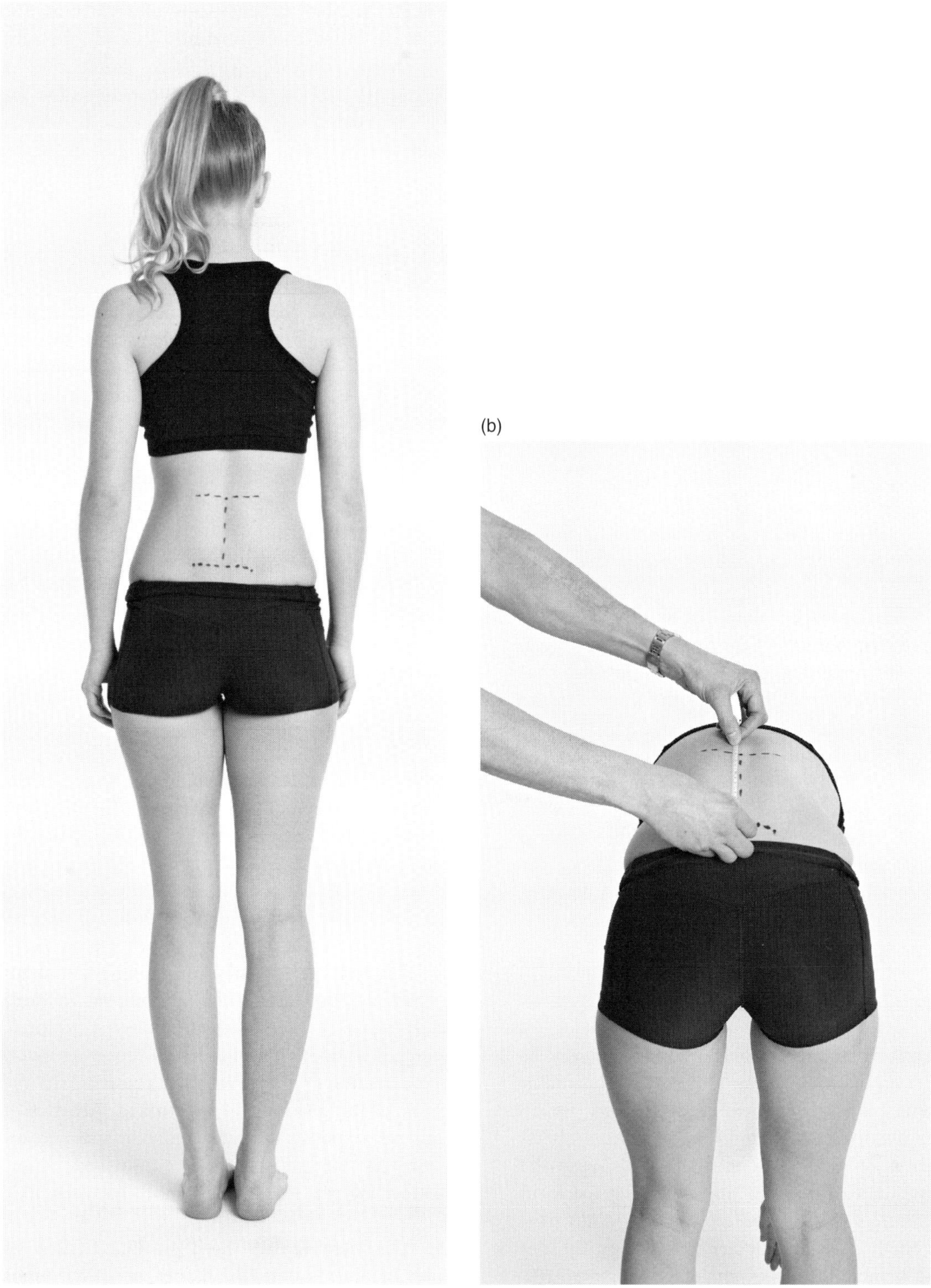

Figure 7.4 **a** Forward flexion of the lumbar spine can be quantified by Schober's test. A 10-cm line is drawn from a point midway between the posterior superior iliac spines. **b** With flexion the length of this line should increase by at least 5 cm in length.

(b)

(a)

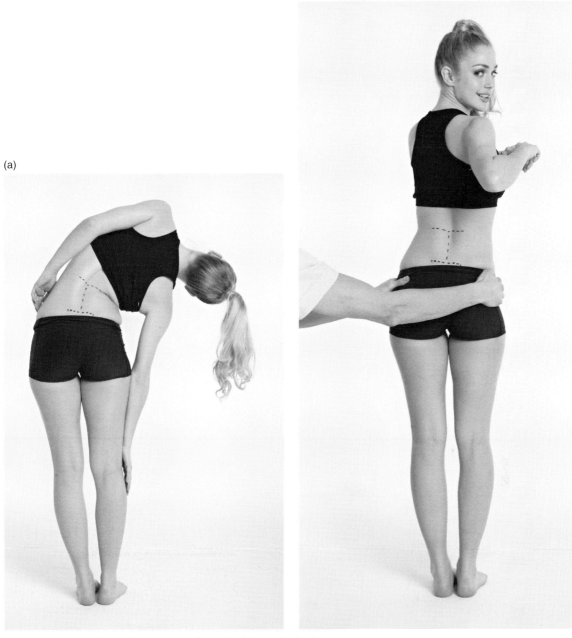

Figure 7.5 a Lateral flexion. **b** Rotation is performed with the pelvis fixed.

(a)

(b)

(c)

(d)

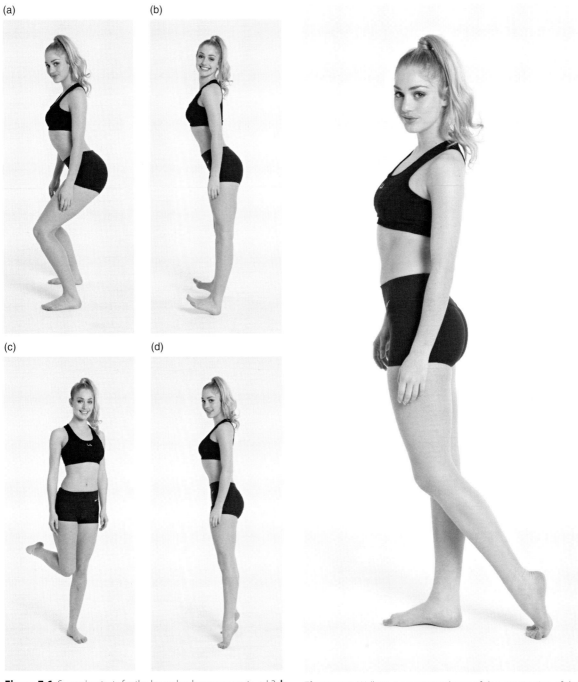

Figure 7.6 Screening tests for the lower lumbar nerve roots. **a** L3; **b** L4; **c** L5; **d** S1.

Figure 7.7 Walking is an essential part of the examination of the cervical, thoracic and lumbar spines.

(b)

(a)

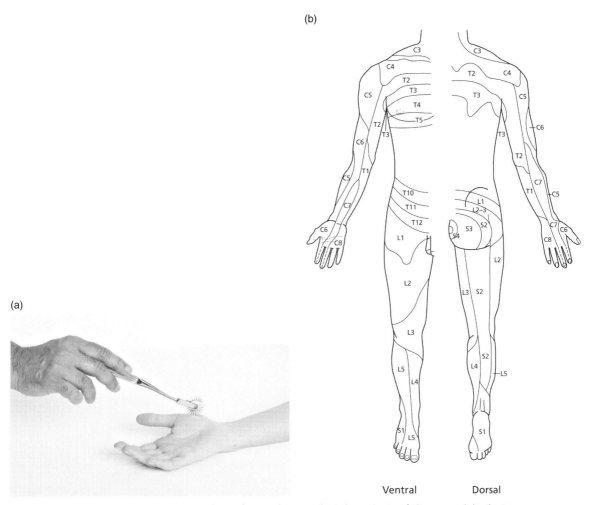

Ventral   Dorsal

Figure 7.8 a Assessing sensation is an essential part of a complete neurological examination. **b** Dermatomal distributions.

Special tests/provocative tests

Cervical spine

Symptoms of cervical radiculopathy can be exacerbated by Spurling's manoeuvre,[7] which narrows the involved neuroforamen. The neck is loaded by axial pressure and then gently hyperextended. It is then laterally flexed and rotated to the side of the suspected lesion (Figure 7.12). Significant relief of symptoms with subsequent abduction of the ipsilateral shoulder (shoulder abduction relief test) lends further support to the diagnosis of intervertebral disc herniation. A positive Tinel's sign can sometimes be elicited over the exiting nerve root.

If there is suspicion of thoracic outlet syndrome (such as pain and paraesthesiae in the arm with overhead activity), then provocative tests for obliteration of the radial pulse or reproduction of symptoms can be performed.[8] In Adson's manoeuvre (Figure 7.13a), the head is extended and rotated to the affected side. The arm is abducted 15° and the radial pulse felt. Obliteration of the pulse with deep inspiration while maintaining the same position is suggestive of thoracic outlet syndrome.[9] Roos[10] described abducting the shoulders and flexing the elbows to 90° (Figure 7.13b). In this position the shoulders are braced backwards and the patient is asked to flex and extend the fingers

Table 7.1a The muscle innervation and reflex values of the upper limb muscles

Action	Principal muscles	Major root values
Shoulder abduction	Supraspinatus/deltoid	C5
Elbow flexion	Brachialis/biceps brachii	C5, C6
Wrist extension	Extensor carpi radialis/ulnaris	C6, C7
Elbow extension	Triceps	C6, C7, C8
Finger extension	Extensor digitorum/pollicis/indicis	C7, C8
Finger flexion	Flexor pollicis/digitorum communis	C8
Finger abduction	Dorsal interossei	C8, T1
Finger adduction	Palmar interossei	C8, T1

Table 7.1b The muscle innervation and reflex values of the lower limb muscles

Action	Principal muscles	Major root values
Hip flexion	Iliopsoas	L1, L2
Hip adduction	Adductor longus/magnus	L2, L3
Knee extension	Quadriceps femoris	L3, L4
Foot dorsiflexion	Tibialis anterior	L4
Toe extension	Extensor digitorum/hallucis	L5
Hip abduction	Gluteus medius/minimis	L4, L5
Hip extension	Gluteus maximus	L5, S1
Knee flexion	Hamstrings	S1
Foot plantar flexion	Gastrocnemius and soleus	S1, S2
Toe flexion	Flexor digitorum/hallucis longus	S1, S2

rapidly. Reproduction of the symptoms is thought to be indicative of thoracic outlet syndrome. Broadly speaking, Adson's manoeuvre assesses the vascular component of a thoracic outlet syndrome and Roos' test assesses the neurological component.

Peripheral nerve entrapments must also be excluded by appropriate tests (discussed in Chapter 6) when numbness, paraesthesia and weakness are reported in the upper limb. Remember also that radiculopathy and peripheral nerve entrapments may coexist and in these cases electromyographs and nerve conduction studies will be required to elucidate the major contributor to the symptoms.

Flexion of the neck that precipitates lightning pains or paraesthesia in the lower limbs represents L'hermitte's sign and is characteristic of cervical spinal myelopathy (Figure 7.14). Other important long tract signs in the assessment of this condition are:

- The plantar responses – when performing this test use a gentle stroke with your thumb nail. The use of the pointed end of a reflex hammer or objects such as a car key is to be avoided

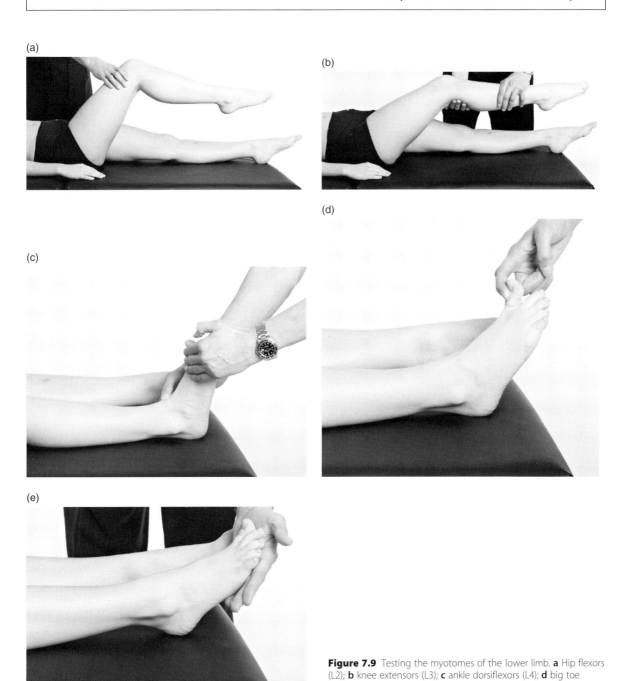

(a)

(b)

(c)

(d)

(e)

Figure 7.9 Testing the myotomes of the lower limb. **a** Hip flexors (L2); **b** knee extensors (L3); **c** ankle dorsiflexors (L4); **d** big toe dorsiflexors (L5); **e** ankle plantarflexors (S1).

- Clonus at the ankle or knee – more than three beats is an abnormal finding
- Hoffman's sign – flick the distal interphalangeal joint of the index or middle finger into flexion and observe the thumb interphalangeal joint. In a positive test this joint will flex (Figure 7.15). A positive test indicates an upper motor neuron lesion
- Inverted radial reflex – finger flexion seen with the brachioradialis tendon reflex

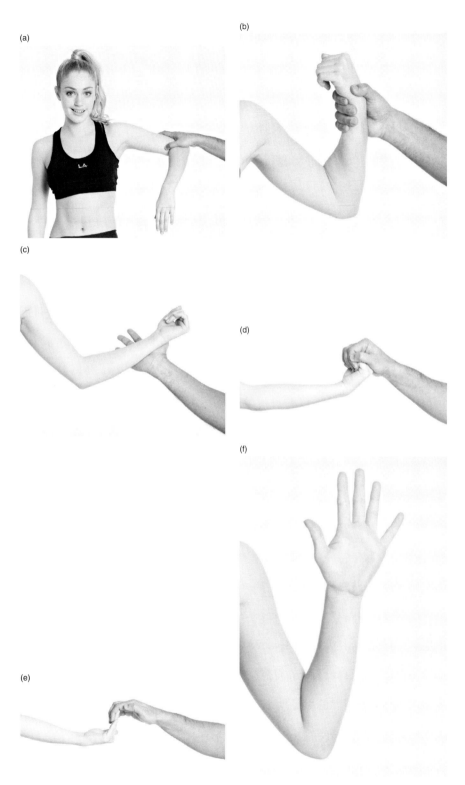

Figure 7.10 Testing the myotomes of the upper limb. **a** Shoulder abductors (C5); **b** elbow flexors (C5,6); **c** elbow extensors (C7,8); **d** wrist flexors and extensors (C6,7); **e** finger flexors and extensors (C7,8); **f** intrinsics of the hand (T1).

(a)

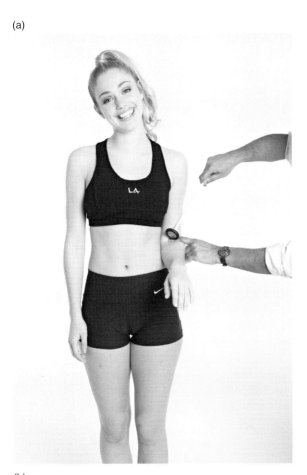

Figure 7.11 **a** Testing the biceps reflex (C5,6). **b** Testing the abdominal reflexes should not be forgotten, especially when examining the thoracic spine.

(b)

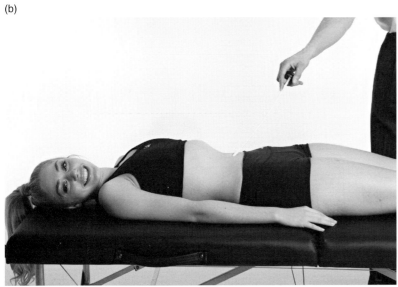

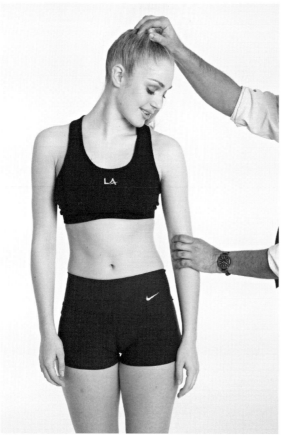

Figure 7.12 Spurling's test, a provocative test for cervical radiculopathy.

- Romberg's test – this assesses the integrity of the dorsal columns. The patient will not be able to maintain a stable stance (with feet together) when asked to close his eyes.

Lumbar spine

Signs of lumbar nerve root irritation, most commonly because of an intervertebral disc protrusion, may be observed when performing a series of tests. These tests rely on reproducing/exacerbating pain in the affected leg and should therefore be performed at the conclusion of the examination and in the order described.

With the patient lying supine slowly raise the affected leg; support it with the palm of the hand under the heel rather than grasping the ankle. Ensure there is no knee flexion. When the patient complains of pain (usually between 30–60° of elevation), stop and ask whether the pain is being experienced in the back or down the leg (Figure 7.16a). This is the straight leg raise test (sciatic stretch test). If the leg is then lowered a little to relieve the discomfort and the foot passively dorsiflexed the pain may be reproduced again (Figure 7.16b). This is Lasègue's sign.[11]

(a)

(b)

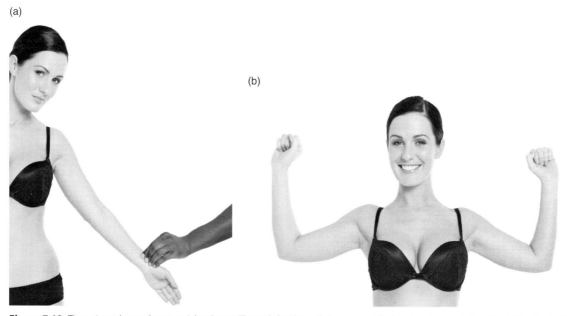

Figure 7.13 Thoracic outlet syndrome. **a** Adson's test. The radial pulse will disappear with deep inspiration. **b** Roos' test. Tingling in the fingers on opening and closing the fists suggests the diagnosis.

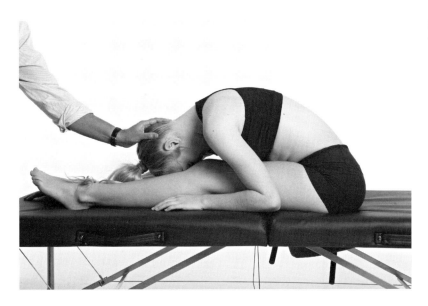

Figure 7.14 L'hermitte's sign. A provocative test for cervical myelopathy. Flexion of the spine results in lightning pains down the legs.

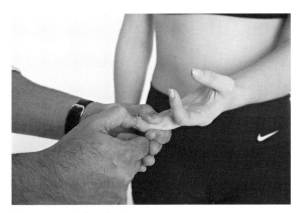

Figure 7.15 Hoffman's sign.

Next, with the knee and hip flexed to 45°, the 'bowstring test' can be carried out by pressing behind the knee over the popliteal nerve with one's thumb. If leg pain is reproduced this indicates sciatic nerve tension (Figure 7.16c). With true sciatic irritation, pressure over the medial or lateral hamstring tendons should not give a positive result.

Finally, with both legs again now flat on the couch and one hand placed gently on the knees to keep them in extension, the patient is asked to sit forward. In the presence of nerve root tension the patient will not be able to sit upright with the knees fully extended.

The 'flip test' is a variation of the last manoeuvre. Sit the patient upright with the knees flexed over the edge of the couch and actively extend the knees in turn (Figure 7.16d). This should produce the same response as the straight leg raise test in the genuine patient.

A straight leg raise test performed on the unaffected leg may give rise to pain in the affected leg – the 'crossover sign'. This has a high sensitivity in diagnosing a prolapsed disc. It has been reported to indicate that the disc protrusion lies in the axilla of the nerve root rather than in the more common lateral position; however, this correlation is not reliable.

Finally, with the patient now lying in the prone position, the femoral stretch test can be performed (Figure 7.16e). With the knee passively flexed to 90° and a hand gently keeping the pelvis against the couch, lift the foot upwards and note the distribution of any pain provoked by this manoeuvre.

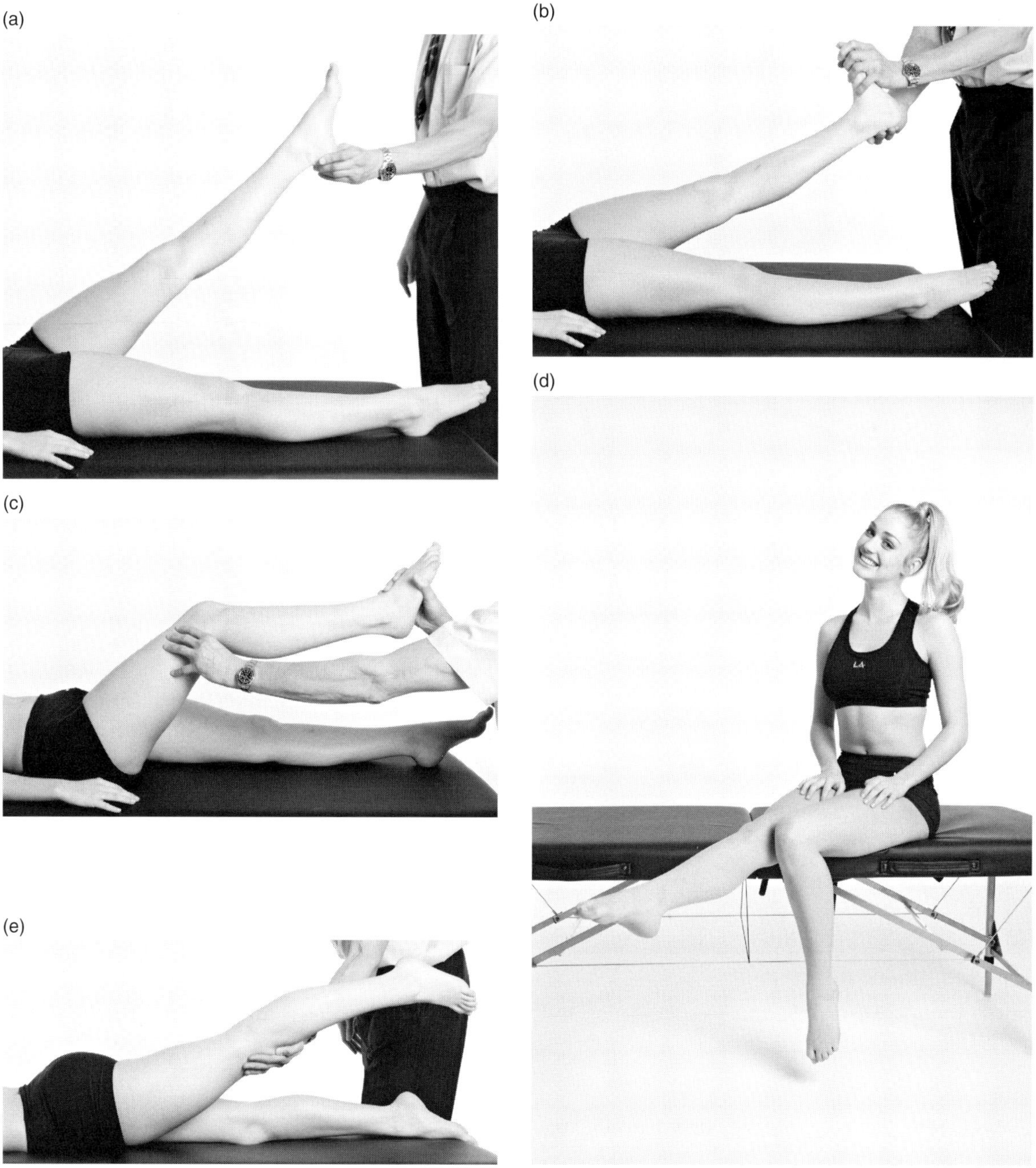

(a)

(b)

(c)

(d)

(e)

Figure 7.16 Provocative tests for lumbar radiculopathy. **a** The straight leg raise test (sciatic stretch). The palm is placed under the heel with the leg extended. Only a reproduction of pain down the leg with elevation is regarded as positive, not an exacerbation of back pain. **b** Lasègue's sign. After lowering the leg, passive dorsiflexion of the ankle increases root tension and reinforces a positive straight leg raise. **c** Bowstring test. The hip and knee is flexed 45° with pressure in the popliteal fossa on the nerve. This increases root tension and results in pain. **d** The flip test. The patient sits upright on the examination couch with the knees flexed over the side. Active extension of the knee resulting in pain down the leg is a positive result as this is equivalent to a straight leg raise test. **e** Femoral stretch test. The hip is extended with the knee extended or flexed. Pain shoots down the front of the thigh in a positive test.

Summary

Summary of examination of the lumbar spine

Step 1
Stand the patient and look

Step 2
Feel

Step 3
Movement
Then tip toe, heel stance, squat and standing on one leg

Step 4
Walk the patient

Step 5
Lie the patient down

- Complete neurological examination. Tone, power, sensation, reflexes
- Provocative tests – straight leg raise, Lasègue's, bowstring, crossover, femoral stretch
- Hip range of movement and peripheral pulses if needed
- (PR)

Stand and look

Clinical examination of the spine starts with standing the patient and looking from the back, assessing any curves, scars and any other stigmata of spinal disease such as café-au-lait spots. Look from the side at any lumbar lordosis and kyphosis as well as cervical spine lordosis. Look from the front.

Feel

Palpate down the bony prominences and paraspinal area of the spinal column.

Move

Movements are forward flexion (quantified by Schober's test), lateral flexion, extension and rotation. Forward flexion is probably the most useful clinically, with lateral flexion and rotation rarely adding much information. Rotation is performed by fixing the pelvis with the examiner's hands or asking the patient to sit and rotate.

Walk

Before walking the patient do a quick screen for the lower lumbar nerve roots by asking the patient to squat and get up (L3), to stand on heels (L4), to stand on one leg, effectively performing Trendelenburg's test (L5) and ask them to stand on tip toes (S1).

Then ask the patient to walk, assessing the gait and looking for any neurological pattern of gait.

Lie patient down

A complete neurological examination is performed, including sensation, tone, power and reflexes.

Tone – passively roll the hips into internal and external rotation.

With regard to the **myotomes**, an easy way to remember the nerve root level for the movements is that all the movements on the anterior aspect of the lower limb are in sequence – hip flexion L2, knee extension L3, ankle dorsiflexion L4, big toe extension L5.

In addition, all the movements on the posterior aspect of the lower limb are essentially S1, i.e. hip extension, knee flexion, ankle plantar flexion and big toe flexion.

Lower limb **reflexes** – knee jerk L3/4 (hamstring jerk L5), ankle jerk S1.

Provocative tests of the lumbar spine are: sciatic stretch test, Lasègue's test, bowstring test, cross sciatic stretch test, femoral stretch test.

Summary of examination of the cervical spine

The process of the cervical spine examination is similar to that for the lumbar spine described above.

Step 1
Stand/sit and look

Step 2
Feel

Step 3
Move
– Include Romberg's test

Step 4
Walk the patient

Step 5
Lie patient down

- Neurological examination – upper and lower limbs
- Provocative tests – Spurling's, L'hermitte's
- (PR)

- Walking is also necessary, as in cervical myelopathy the lower limb may be affected
- Neurological examination should include both the upper and lower limbs (for cervical myelopathy). Assess tone, sensation, power, reflexes
- **Myotomes**: shoulder abduction C4/5; elbow flexion C6; elbow extension C7; wrist flexion and extension C6/7; finger flexion and extension C7/8; spread the fingers T1
- **Reflexes**: biceps jerk (C5), brachioradialis reflex (C6), triceps jerk (C7)
- Hoffman's test for upper motor neuron lesions
- Provocative tests include Spurling's test for radicular pain and L'hermitte's manoeuvre for cervical myelopathy.

References

1   Fairbank CJT, Davies JB, Couper J, O'Brien JP. The Oswestry low back pain disability questionnaire. *Physiotherapy* 1980;**66**:271–273.

2   Ware JE Jr, Snow KK, Kosinski M, Gandek B. *SF-36 Health Survey; Manual and Interpretation Guide.* Boston: The Health Institute, 1993.

3   Waddell G, McCulloch JA, Kummel E, Venner RM. Nonorganic physical signs in low-back pain. *Spine* 1980;**5**:107–112.

4   Schober P. Lendenwirbelsaule und Kreuzschmerzen. *Munch Med Wschr* 1937;**84**:336.

5   Macrea IF, Wright V. Measurement of back movement. *Ann Rheum Dis* 1969;**28**:584–593.

6   Medical Research Council. *Aids to the Examination of the Peripheral Nervous System.* London: Medical Research Council, 1976.

7   Spurling RG. *Lesions of the Cervical Intevertebral Disc.* Springfield: Thomas, 1956.

8   Oates SD, Daley RA. Thoracic outlet syndrome. *Hand Clin* 1996;**12**:705–718.

9   Adson W, Coffey JR. Cervical rib: a method of anterior approach for relief of symptoms by division of the scalenus anticus. *Ann Surg* 1927;**85**:839–855.

10 Roos D. Transaxillary approach for first rib resection to relieve thoracic outlet syndrome. *Ann Surg* 1966;**163**:354–358.

11 Lasègue C. Considerations sur la sciatique. *Arch Gen Med* 1864;**2**:558.

Examination of the hip

Ian Stockley, Richard Villar and Alexandra Dimitrakopoulou

History

A detailed clinical history and complete physical examination are mandatory in the assessment of the patient with a painful hip. Often a tentative diagnosis can be made on the history alone. The onset (acute or insidious), duration and severity of symptoms, as well as any earlier injury, are significant in any history taken. Examination and subsequent investigations allow for confirmation or modification of the presumptive diagnosis.

Presenting complaints in hip pathology may include pain, limp and stiffness. Patients may not complain of stiffness per se but of the disability produced by it (e.g. the inability to put socks on). In trying to evaluate a patient's symptomatology it is important to know what effect, if any, the symptoms have on the patient's ability to undertake activities of everyday living. Mechanical symptoms such as locking, clicking, catching or popping can also be presenting symptoms in their own right.

It is important to ask patients whether they have had any previous problems with their hips. Childhood conditions affecting the hip may cause symptoms in early adult life because of the development of secondary degenerative changes. In addition, a history of previous surgery is very important when contemplating further surgical procedures as consideration needs to be given to previous scars, the surgical approach, skeletal deformity and, in addition, the increased risk of infection with arthroplasty surgery.

Several validated hip assessment scores are now available, and these allow for a more objective assessment of hip function. The Harris hip score is scored by the examiner and emphasizes range of motion, pain and function. The Oxford hip score and the WOMAC Osteoarthritis Index are scored by the patient and so remove any potential clinician bias. These scores, if readministered after treatment, are useful in objectively quantifying both how patients perceive the results of that treatment modality and whether it led to improved wellbeing and functional ability.

The patient's individual occupational and recreational demands need to be known when discussing management options. What is appropriate for one patient may not be so for another, despite initial similarities.

Pain

Pain in the groin or thigh region is most likely a result of hip disease and is believed to arise from the joint capsule, synovial lining and labrum. Radiation to the anterior, medial or lateral thigh is common, as is pain referred to the knee. Obviously, patients may have symptoms related to the knees as a direct consequence of knee pathology, but referred pain from above always needs to be considered. A common symptom of intra-articular soft tissue pathology is the so-called 'C' sign, where the patient demonstrates the location of their pain by cupping the lateral aspect of the hip in their hand, fingers anteriorly and thumb posteriorly.[1] 'Hip pain' localized to the gluteal region is often referred pain from lumbosacral pathology and there may be associated radicular symptoms and signs. Differentiation between hip and back pain can usually be made on the basis of history, clinical examination and X-rays, but, if in doubt, an injection of local anaesthetic into the hip joint can be very useful. The presence of inguinal herniae, or the so-called 'sportsman's groin',

Examination Techniques in Orthopaedics, Second Edition, ed. Nick Harris and Fazal Ali. Published by Cambridge University Press. © Cambridge University Press 2014.

produces groin symptoms that may be increased by coughing, sneezing and the Valsalva manoeuvre.

Pain as a consequence of arthritis is usually exacerbated by exercise and relieved by rest. However, as the pathology progresses, pain at rest becomes a feature.

The differential diagnosis of a patient presenting with hip pain should always include infection. Pyogenic infection of the hip presents as pain localized to the groin or inner thigh. Pain secondary to infection is constant and unrelenting in character. The patient will experience pain with weightbearing but will also have pain at rest. When pain is caused by haematogenous spread, the onset is often acute and caused by distension of the joint capsule and secondary muscle spasm. A more insidious onset is the norm when the infection is by direct extension, as there is no dramatic increase in intra-articular pressure.

Claudication-like pain may also be present in degenerative hip pathology, and a differential diagnosis should consider neurogenic (presence of stenosis of the spinal canal) or vascular (presence of peripheral vascular disease) causes. With neurogenic causes, when the patient bends forward, the pain decreases. Meanwhile, with a vascular cause the patient reports distal rather than proximal pain and needs to sit for a while.

Stiffness and limp

Patients do not often complain of stiffness but complain of the difficulties they have undertaking activities of everyday living as a consequence of the stiffness, i.e. going up stairs, cutting toe nails and putting on socks, etc. The term stiffness usually includes some loss of range of motion; it is a feeling experienced by the patient.

Limping can result from a variety of reasons, including pain, limb length inequality, muscle weakness and bone and joint deformity. If the hip is very stiff then patients often complain of a limp and not necessarily pain.

Snapping and clicking hips

Snapping and clicking hips tend to occur in adolescents and young adults.[2] Patients often produce the symptoms and demonstrate the physical signs on demand and so these tend to become habitual in nature. Intra-articular and extra-articular

pathologies have been described, although often there is no obvious abnormality detected either clinically or by investigation. Pain can be associated with the mechanical symptoms and radiates to the groin or laterally towards the greater trochanter area.

Examination
General

Examination starts as soon as the patient walks into the room. Is a cane or crutches needed? Is there a limp? Is he or she in pain? Often there are many clues, which can be explored later during the formal examination.

Inspection

With the patient standing barefoot and dressed down to underwear, muscle wasting and scars can be seen and posture is noted for the presence of contractures, spinal deformity and the ability to stand with feet flat on the ground (Figure 8.1). A leg length discrepancy may now be seen and, if present, could be assessed at this stage by asking the patient to stand on blocks of wood of varying height. The patient is asked 'Do you feel level now?' and the blocks are changed as necessary until the patient feels level. This is probably a better assessment of leg length inequality than using a tape measure as the patient is actively involved in this assessment and it is how he or she feels when standing that is important rather than a measurement on a tape measure. Looking and palpating the iliac crests gives an assessment of pelvic obliquity, which will be corrected if the obliquity is caused by leg length inequality. However, fixed obliquity resulting from lumbosacral disease cannot be compensated for in this manner.

Trendelenburg's test

Hip abductor function can be assessed by the Trendelenburg test. In 1895 Trendelenburg recorded observations describing the gait of patients with congenitally dislocated hips (CDH). He described how the upper body swings to the side of weightbearing in a child with CDH. Later he went on to describe the pelvic inclination on single leg weightbearing, which became known as the Trendelenburg sign. This was originally described with the examiner standing behind the patient so that the dimples

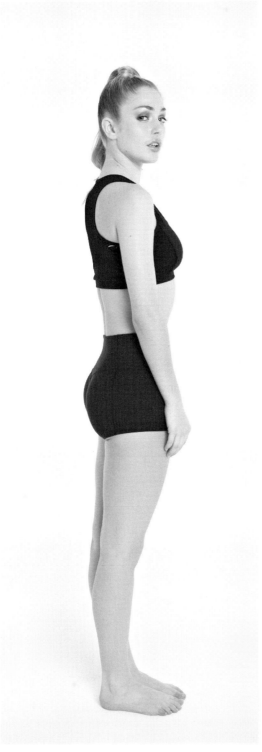

Figure 8.1 Stand the patient and look from the front, side and back. Observe the spine and knees to see if he or she is compensating for hip pathology.

overlying the posterior superior iliac spines could be seen to move up and down when the test was being performed.

It is our experience, however, that unless somebody is actually facing the patient, he or she is reluctant to stand on one leg, particularly if the hip is painful. When assessing the patient, ask the patient to face the examiner and then ask him or her to place their forearms on the examiner's, thereby giving support and, hopefully, a feeling of confidence. The patient is then asked to stand on one leg and bend the opposite knee to 90° without flexing the hip. This action eliminates the role of hip flexors as they play a role in pelvic stability and may affect the Trendelenburg sign (Figure 8.2). The test is then repeated by standing on the other leg. The sign is deemed negative, i.e. the abductor mechanism is normal, when the pelvis remains level. A positive result indicates abductor mechanism dysfunction and the pelvis on the unsupported side will descend. A patient standing on his right leg would be Trendelenburg-positive for the right if the left side dipped.

A Trendelenburg test can be positive for two main reasons: neurological or mechanical. Neurological causes can result from generalized motor weakness as seen with myelomeningocele and spinal cord lesions or more specific problems, e.g. superior gluteal nerve dysfunction. The mechanical group includes conditions that affect the abductor muscle lever arm (e.g. CDH, coxa vara and fractures). These conditions shorten the length of the muscle from its origin to its insertion and significantly weaken its strength.

It is important to be aware that patients who have a weakened abductor mechanism may not descend on one side when assessing for the Trendelenburg sign, as they can compensate by leaning over the affected hip to shift the body's centre of gravity in that direction. This is called a Trendelenburg lurch. However, patients with advanced arthritis of the hip may lurch towards the ipsilateral stance limb simply because the arthritis prevents the pelvic tilt and, to maintain balance, the patient leans over.

The delayed Trendelenburg sign is really non-specific. Any painful hip condition will be positive after the patient has been performing the test for 30 seconds to a minute. We question its value.

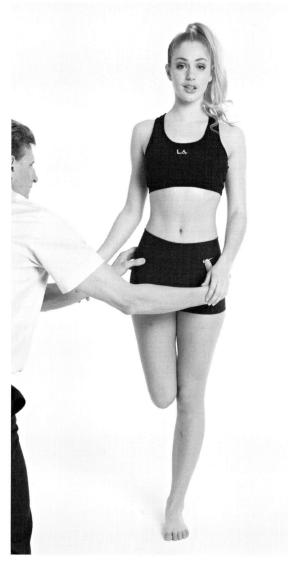

Figure 8.2 Trendelenburg test – the surgeon faces the patient and asks him or her to stand on one leg. The opposite knee is flexed behind to 90°. The pelvis should remain level or rise. A positive result is when the pelvis dips on the unsupported side.

Gait

Abnormal pathology in the lower limb is often demonstrated by changes in the gait pattern, whether it is a compensatory adaptation to pain, loss of motion or weakness (Figure 8.3).

Common gait patterns include:

- **Antalgic gait**: pain in the hip on weightbearing can be diminished by reducing the time spent on the affected leg (stance phase) and by leaning the trunk over to the symptomatic side when in stance

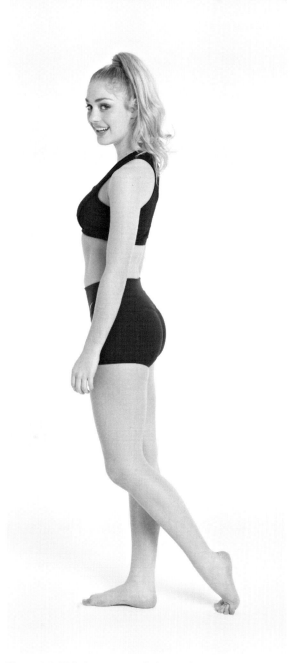

Figure 8.3 Walk the patient and observe the gait.

phase. It also involves an excessive drop in the centre of gravity as a means of reducing peak loading on weightbearing. This produces an uneven stance period, which is the characteristic feature of an antalgic gait.

- **Short-leg gait**: this involves excessive shift of the centre of gravity toward the short side, with a drop of the centre of gravity. It differs from the antalgic gait in that the stance period is equal.
- **Trendelenburg gait**: this is indicated by a drop of the pelvis on the opposite side to the stance limb. However, to maintain centre of gravity above the stance limb it is not unusual for the trunk to lurch towards the ipsilateral stance limb.
- **Gluteus maximus gait**: hip extensor weakness (gluteus maximus) necessitates a forward thrust of the pelvis and backward thrust of the trunk. This position places the centre of gravity posterior to the hip, tenses the iliofemoral ligament and stabilizes the situation.

Supine examination of the hip

As a preliminary step it is important to set the pelvis square (Figure 8.4). Determine from the position of the anterior superior iliac spines whether or not the pelvis is lying square with the limbs. One way of demonstrating this is to ensure that the line between both anterior superior iliac spines is perpendicular to the side of the couch. If it is not, an attempt is made to set it square. If the pelvis cannot be squared up, then there is a fixed adduction or abduction deformity at one or both hips. This should be noted.

Palpation

The hip joint is too deep to assess for the presence of an effusion or synovial thickening. Bony landmarks can be palpated and include the anterior superior iliac spine, the ischial tuberosity and the greater trochanter.

Hip movements

Active and passive movements of the hips should be recorded. Measurements should include flexion and extension, abduction and adduction, internal and external rotation both in flexion and extension. There is considerable variation in the 'normal' range of motion among individuals. The patient with hip pathology may well have significant reduction in movement secondary to pain, bony abnormalities and degenerative changes. The accurate determination of hip movements needs care as restriction of hip movement is easily masked by movement of the pelvis. It is therefore essential to place one hand on the contralateral hemipelvis while the other supports and moves the leg.

Thomas's test

Contracture of the joint capsule will cause deformity. Fixed flexion, fixed adduction and external rotation are the common deformities.[3] A fixed flexion deformity is best determined by performing Thomas's test (Figure 8.5a). Hugh Owen Thomas described this test in 1876. A patient with a fixed flexion deformity at the

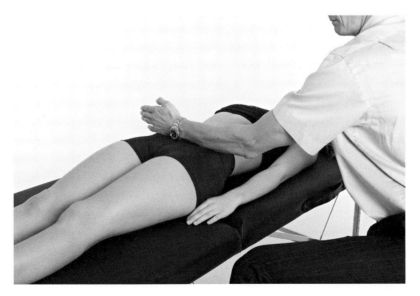

Figure 8.4 Lie the patient on the couch and square the pelvis.

(a)

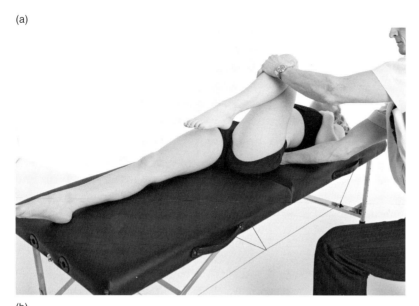

(b)

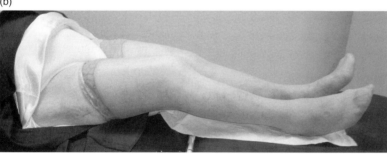

Figure 8.5 a Thomas's test for a flexion deformity of the hip. The hand placed under the lumbar spine confirms that the lumbar lordosis has been eliminated. Any persistent elevation or flexion of the thigh relative to the examination couch represents the flexion deformity. **b** This patient has a fixed flexion deformity of her right hip and is unable to place her leg flat on the bed unless she compensates by increasing her lumbar lordosis.

hip will compensate, when lying on his or her back, by arching the spine and pelvis into an exaggerated lordosis. A hand placed under the back will assess the lumbar lordosis. If the hip not being measured is flexed to its limit, the pelvis rotates and the lordosis is eliminated. During this manoeuvre the other hip, if in fixed flexion, is passively lifted from the couch. The angle through which it is raised is the fixed flexion deformity (Figure 8.5b). An alternative way of assessing fixed flexion deformity is to start with both hips in the knee–chest position. Each hip can be extended separately and the angle from the horizontal to the thigh is the flexion deformity.

Flexion

Hip flexion is normally tested in the supine position with the knee flexed to prevent hamstring tightness restricting movement (Figure 8.6). In the normal hip, flexion is limited by the soft tissues of the thigh and abdomen. Tilt of the pelvis increasing the range of

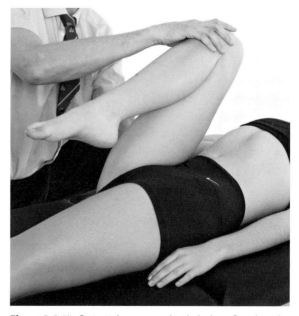

Figure 8.6 Hip flexion is best assessed with the knee flexed to relax the hamstrings.

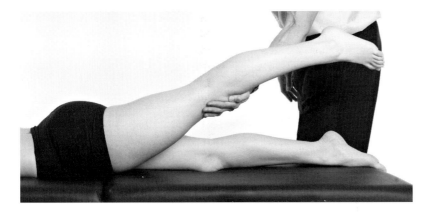

Figure 8.7 Hip extension. This is best performed in the prone position.

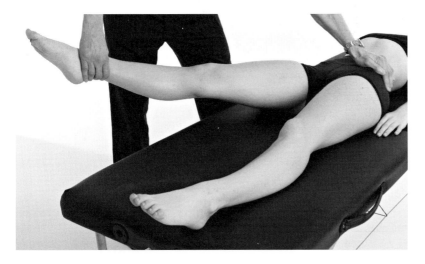

Figure 8.8 Hip abduction. The pelvis is stabilized by the examiner's hand. This is followed by hip adduction.

flexion is best detected by grasping the crest of the ilium. Normal flexion is recorded from 0° to between 100° and 135°.

The primary flexor of the hip is the iliopsoas muscle. Muscle power is assessed by having the patient sitting on the edge of the examination couch with the legs dangling down. The patient is then asked to raise the thigh from the table. The examiner places his hands on the distal thigh and assesses muscle power.

Extension

Extension is best measured in the prone position with the knee either flexed or straight (Figure 8.7). Maximum extension is achieved when the pelvis begins to rotate. The normal range is reported to be from 0° to between 15° and 30°. Extension, especially in the older arthritic patient, is not routinely tested.

The main hip extensor muscle is gluteus maximus, with contributions from the hamstrings. Power of gluteus maximus is best assessed by asking the patient to lift the leg off the couch with the knee flexed. This minimizes the effect of the hamstring muscles.

Abduction

Hip abduction is measured with the patient lying supine and the pelvis stabilized with the examiner's hand on the opposite anterior superior iliac spine (Figure 8.8). Normal ranges are from 0° to between 40° and 45°. False abduction is detected when the contralateral anterior superior iliac spine moves.

Abductor strength is assessed by one hand stabilizing the pelvis while the other applies resistance to the lateral thigh as the patient abducts. Alternatively, with the patient lying on the side, he or she can be asked to abduct against resistance. Flexing the knee relaxes the iliotibial band and isolates the abductors. An abduction deformity is present when the angle

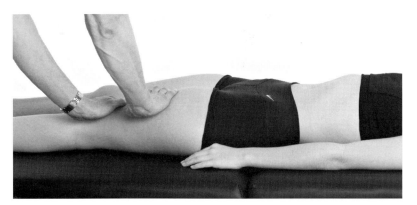

Figure 8.9 Hip rotation in extension.

between the transverse axis of the pelvis and the limb is greater than 90°.

Abduction in flexion is often the first movement to be restricted in osteoarthritis of the hip. The patient flexes his or her hips and knees by drawing the heels towards the buttocks. The knees are then allowed to fall away towards the couch. The normal range is approximately 70°.

Adduction

True adduction can only be measured if the contralateral leg is in a position of abduction. If it is in a neutral position, then a degree of pelvic tilt comes into play as the examined leg crosses over the contralateral static leg. Hip adduction is measured with the patient lying supine and, as with abduction, the pelvis needs to be stabilized when measuring the range of movement. Normal ranges are from 0° to between 20° and 30°.

Adductor strength is measured by resisting adduction of the abducted leg in the supine position. The examining hand is placed on the medial side of the knee. Alternatively, in the lateral position the patient can be asked to adduct against resistance.

An adduction deformity is seen when the angle between the transverse axis of the pelvis and the limb is less than 90°.

Rotation in extension (Figure 8.9)

Internal rotation is considered normal if the hip rotates from 0° to between 30° and 40°. External rotation is slightly greater and is recorded from 0° to between 40° and 60°. It is preferable to use an imaginary line from the patella, as opposed to the foot, to act as a pointer for measurement. Alternatively, rotational movements can be measured with

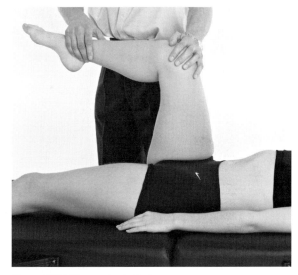

Figure 8.10 Hip rotation in flexion.

the patient lying prone with the hip extended and the knee flexed at 90°.

Rotation in flexion (Figure 8.10)

Early signs of hip pathology (e.g. an irritable hip) can be picked up by evaluating rotation in flexion. External rotation is usually greater except in cases of excessive femoral neck anteversion. The range for internal rotation is from 0° to between 30° and 40°, with external rotation from 0° to between 40° and 50°.

Measurements of leg length

It is important to know whether any leg length inequality present is real or apparent. Although it is usually necessary to measure for true discrepancy it is not so for apparent inequality, unless there is fixed

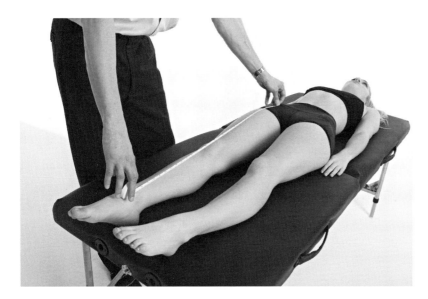

Figure 8.11 Real leg length measurements. The unaffected side is placed in the same position as the affected.

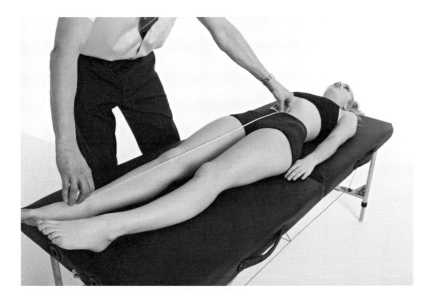

Figure 8.12 Apparent leg length measurements are taken from the medial malleolus to a midline structure such as the umbilicus.

pelvic obliquity. Ideally it would be best to measure from the centre of the femoral head, the normal axis of hip movement. However, as there is no surface landmark then the nearest fixed point, the anterior superior iliac spine, is chosen. Distally, **real leg length** measurements are taken to the medial malleolus (Figure 8.11). If there is a fixed deformity, the good leg must be placed in a comparably deformed position relative to the pelvis before measurements are taken. If not, measurements will be inaccurate as the angle between the leg and pelvis will be different on the two sides. For this reason it is better to assess leg length

measurements after hip movements and any fixed deformities are noted.

Apparent shortening is measured from any midline point in the body, e.g. umbilicus, xiphisternum (Figure 8.12). Adduction makes the limb appear shorter – each 10° of fixed adduction adds a further 3 cm of apparent shortening to any real shortening that the disorder may have caused.

Is the shortening above or below the knee? If both knees are flexed while the heels remain together on the couch, it can be seen whether shortening is in the femur or tibia (Figure 8.13). This is called Galeazzi's test.

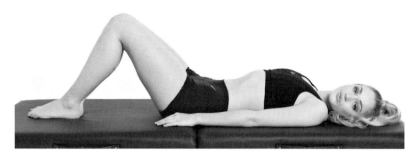

Figure 8.13 Galeazzi's test. Placing both heels together on the examination couch allows the examiner to determine whether a leg length discrepancy is above or below the knee. Tibial shortening causes the affected knee to lie lower than the unaffected side. Femoral shortening causes the knee to adopt a more proximal position.

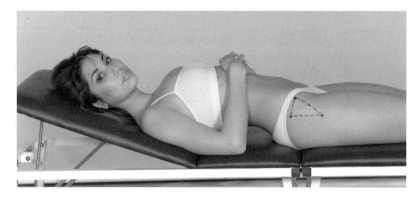

Figure 8.14 Bryant's triangle.

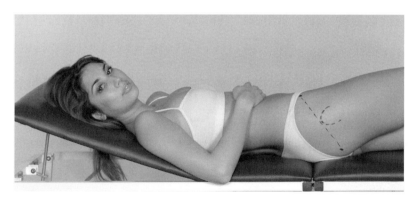

Figure 8.15 Nelaton's line. The greater trochanter should lie on or below a line connecting the anterior superior iliac spine and the ischial tuberosity.

Having determined that the limb length inequality is in the femur, is it above the trochanter (suggesting a problem in or near the hip joint) or below the trochanter? X-rays would obviously tell the answer but there are clinical measurements that can be taken. However, in everyday clinical practice they are not often used. The tests described for shortening above the greater trochanter include Bryant's triangle, Nelaton's line and Schoemaker's line.

Bryant's triangle

With the patient lying supine, a perpendicular is dropped from the anterior superior spine of the ilium; this meets a second line projected upwards from the tip of the greater trochanter. The length of this second line is compared between the two sides (Figure 8.14). Relative shortening on one side indicates that the femur is displaced upwards as a consequence of a problem in or near the hip joint. If the pathology is bilateral, Bryant's triangle is not helpful.

Nelaton's line

The patient lies with the affected side uppermost. A tape measure or string is stretched from the ischial tuberosity to the anterior iliac spine (Figure 8.15). Normally the greater trochanter lies on or below the line and so if the trochanter lies above the line, the femur has been displaced proximally.

Schoemaker's line

A line is projected on each side of the body from the greater trochanter through and beyond the anterior superior iliac spine. Normally the two lines meet in the midline above the umbilicus. If there is a proximal femoral problem the lines will meet away from the midline on the opposite side. If the problem is bilateral the lines will meet at or near the midline but below the umbilicus.

Soft tissue evaluation of the hip

Log-roll test

The log-roll test evaluates hip joint pain simply by moving the femoral head in relation to the acetabulum and the joint capsule. The patient lies supine and the examiner places his or her hands on the limb, gently rolling the hip into internal and external rotation. A positive test elicits pain but its absence does not exclude the hip as a source of symptoms.

Capsular laxity and instability of the hip can also be assessed with this test. The examiner rolls the leg from internal to external rotation and then lets the leg rest in whatever position it naturally adopts. The test is positive when there is no obvious endpoint and the affected limb lies in more external rotation than the unaffected side. This indicates possible laxity of the iliofemoral ligament.

Impingement tests

The **anterior impingement test** (also known as the anterior femoroacetabular impingement test) is a useful and more sensitive test to reveal any

intra-articular hip pathology, in particular a torn acetabular labrum. With the patient supine, the hip is flexed to 90°, then adducted and internally rotated (Figure 8.16). A positive test reproduces the patient's pain in the groin. A positive test may sometimes be accompanied by a clicking or popping feeling.

Similarly, the **DEXTRIT** (Dynamic EXTernal Rotation Impingement Test) may reproduce a patient's pain. The patient lies supine and the examined hip is flexed beyond 90° and then passively abducted and externally rotated.

A **posterior impingement test** is useful to identify any conflict between the posterior acetabular wall and the femoral neck. For this test, the patient lies supine at the edge of the examination couch with the affected leg dangling. The contralateral leg is held in flexion while the examiner fully extends the affected hip while abducting and externally rotating the leg (Figure 8.17).

The **Patrick** or **FABER (Flexion, ABduction, External Rotation) test** may be used to differentiate pathology within the sacroiliac joint from pain arising from the posterior aspect of the hip.[4] It is also a valuable test for posterior impingement. The patient lies supine, placing their ipsilateral foot on the contralateral knee. This is the so-called Figure-4 position. The ipsilateral leg is then allowed to relax and the leg will be seen to drop outwards to a variable degree. When the endpoint of this manoeuvre has been reached, the examiner places one hand on the flexed knee and the other on the anterior superior iliac spine of the contralateral side and presses gently

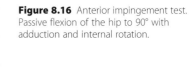

Figure 8.16 Anterior impingement test. Passive flexion of the hip to 90° with adduction and internal rotation.

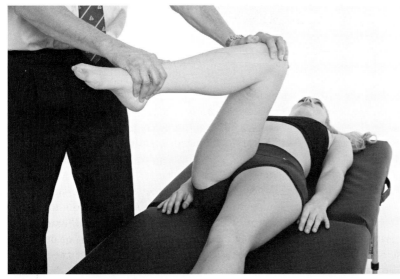

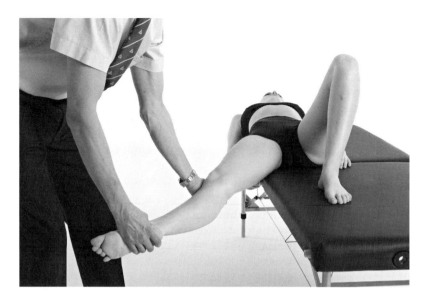

Figure 8.17 Posterior impingement test. The patient is positioned at the edge of the examination table and passive extension, abduction and external rotation of the hip is performed.

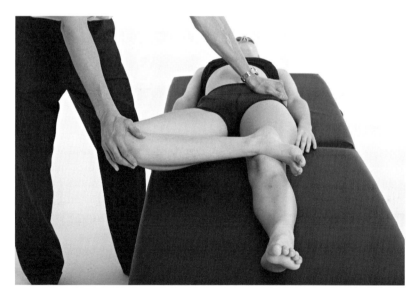

Figure 8.18 The Patrick (FABER) test. The patient lies supine while placing the ipsilateral foot on the contralateral knee, the Figure-4 position. The examiner places one hand on the flexed knee and the other on the anterior superior iliac spine of the contralateral side and presses gently downwards on the flexed knee.

downwards on the flexed knee (Figure 8.18). Increased pain can be elicited but with different localization of symptoms for the sacroiliac joint and posterior hip. The test is performed bilaterally.

The FABER distance is measured for both legs as the vertical distance between the knee and the examination table. It will be reduced in the presence of posterior hip impingement

The **ischiofemoral impingement test** is sometimes referred to as the HEADER (Hip Extension, ADduction, External Rotation) test. Ischiofemoral impingement is caused by abnormal contact between the ischium and the lesser trochanter of the femur. The patient is positioned supine, the ipsilateral knee is flexed to 90° and the hip is then extended, adducted and externally rotated. A positive test elicits pain deep within the groin and/or medial aspect of the buttock.

Tests of hip contractures

Ely's test is used to evaluate a tight rectus femoris. The patient lies prone and the knee is passively flexed. If the rectus femoris is contracted, then the patient's hip, on the same side as the flexed knee, will

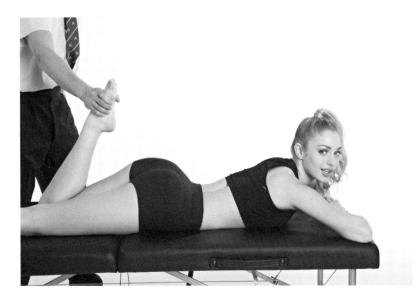

Figure 8.19 Ely's test. Passive flexion of the knee in the presence of a tight rectus femoris leads to the ipsilateral buttock rising.

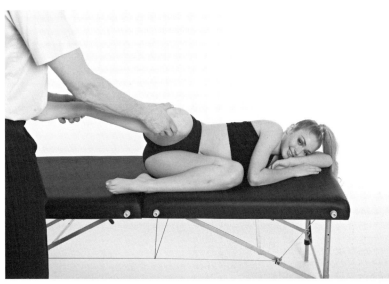

Figure 8.20 Ober's test. The patient lies on the unaffected side. The affected hip is flexed and abducted 45°. This hip is then slowly extended. Normally in bringing the hip into extension it will be possible to adduct the hip to the midline. In the presence of a tight iliotibial band the leg remains abducted.

spontaneously rise. Normally the hip will remain flat against the examination couch (Figure 8.19).

Ober's test evaluates contracture of the fascia lata or iliotibial band. The patient lies on the unaffected side. The unaffected hip is maximally flexed to flatten the lumbar spine. The affected hip is flexed and abducted 45° (Figure 8.20). This hip is then slowly extended. Normally, in bringing the hip into extension it will be possible to adduct the hip to the midline. If the leg remains abducted this is indicative of a contracture of the iliotibial band.

Phelps' test evaluates tightness in the gracilis muscle. The patient lies supine and the affected hip

is abducted as far as possible. The knee is then flexed over the side of the couch (Figure 8.21). If more abduction is possible by flexing the knee (and relaxing the gracilis), then this signifies that the gracilis is tight.

Other tests

Iliopsoas tendon snapping (coxa saltans interna)

On occasion the iliopsoas tendon can snap over the anterior capsule or iliopectineal eminence during hip movements. To identify this, the examiner brings the ipsilateral hip from flexion, abduction and external rotation into extension and internal rotation. The test

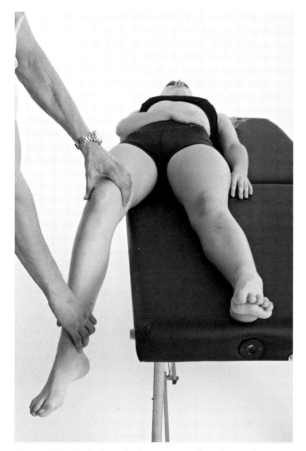

Figure 8.21 Phelps' test. In the presence of a tight gracilis, further abduction of the hip is possible on flexion of the knee.

is positive when there is an audible click or clunk, which can sometimes be painful.

Straight leg raise against resistance

This is also known as the Stinchfield test. It is an assessment of iliopsoas strength and also a sign of intra-articular pathology as the iliopsoas presses against the acetabular labrum during active resistance. The patient performs an active straight leg raise to 45° and is asked to resist as the examiner pushes downward on the affected leg. A positive test is noted when pain is elicited or weakness of iliopsoas identified.

Piriformis test

The piriformis test evaluates pathology within the piriformis muscle itself or irritation of the sciatic nerve by the muscle's margin. The patient lies on his or her side with the affected side uppermost. The hip is then flexed to 45° and the knee to 90°. With one hand the examiner stabilizes the pelvis and

with the other adducts the flexed hip. This manoeuvre stretches the piriformis muscle. Localized pain over the piriformis muscle suggests tendonitis but, when the pain is along the course of the sciatic nerve, this may be an indication of entrapment of the sciatic nerve by the piriformis muscle itself.

Neurovascular examination

Finally, having examined the hip, it is important to carry out a vascular and neurological examination of the whole limb.

Summary

Summary of hip examination
Step 1 Stand the patient and look
Step 2 Trendelenburg test
Step 3 Walk the patient
Step 4 Lie patient down and square the pelvis
Step 5 Thomas's test then range of movement
Step 6 Leg length measurement
Step 7 Special tests Impingement: anterior impingement test, posterior impingement test and FABER test. Contractures: Ely's test, Ober's test, Phelps' test.

Stand and look

Expose the patient adequately, remembering to lift the underwear and looking closely for any scars. Look at the general attitude of the lower limb. Look from the front, side, both laterally and medially and behind. In particular, when looking from the side assess the degree of lumbar lordosis and when looking from behind looking for any associated scoliosis. The lumbar lordosis may indicate any fixed flexion deformity of the hip and a scoliosis may help to indicate a leg length discrepancy.

Trendelenburg's test

In performing Trendelenburg's test, flexion should occur only at the knee. Demonstrate this to the patient. It is reassuring to hold on to the patient's waist and ask them to hold on to your shoulder or forearm as many older patients may have difficulty balancing on one leg.

Walk

Whilst the patient is walking it is important to comment on the gait. Knowledge of the stages of the gait cycle will help in this. Remember to look for walking aids.

Lie patient down

Make sure the couch is flat and square the pelvis. Squaring the pelvis is very important as all assessments of deformities and leg length should be based on a squared pelvis. By squaring the pelvis we mean that both anterior superior iliac spines are perpendicular to the side of the examination couch.

Thomas's test

Thomas's test is performed to assess fixed flexion deformity of the hip. What it is actually achieving is obliterating the lumbar spine compensation that takes place when a patient has fixed flexion deformity of the hip. As such, it gives the true measurement of the fixed flexion deformity. Up to 30° degrees of fixed flexion deformity of the hip can be compensated by increasing lumbar lordosis.

Movements

First, ask the patient to actively flex the affected hip as far as it will go, and then passively take it beyond that point to see the full degree of flexion of the hip. Then perform other movements: abduction, adduction, internal rotation and external rotation.

Rotation both in flexion and extension is especially important in the young patient as it may give an indication of an abnormally shaped femoral head.

Leg length measurements

Note that it is important to assess the contralateral hip movements prior to proceeding with leg length measurements as both limbs need to be placed in exactly the same degree of deformity for the measurements to be accurate.

Real and apparent lengths are measured and these can be fine tuned by doing Galeazzi's test to assess whether shortening is above or below the knee. Bryant's triangle or Nelaton's line will make clear whether the femoral shortening is above or below the trochanter.

Then, if necessary, stand the patient and perform the block test (see page 122).

Special tests

These are mainly for soft tissue pathology. There are many described but the important ones are indicated above in the Summary box.

References

1   Byrd JW. Physical examination. In: Byrd JW. Ed. *Operative Hip Arthroscopy*. New York: Springer, 2005, pp.36–50.

2   Beals RK. Painful snapping hip in young adults. *West J Med* 1993;**159**:481–482.

3   Thurston A. Assessment of fixed flexion deformity of the hip. *Clin Orthop* 1982;**169**:186–189.

4   Broadhurst N, Bond M. Pain provocation tests for the assessment of sacroiliac joint dysfunction. *J Spin Disorders* 1998;**11**:341–345.

Examination of the knee

Fazal Ali and Derek Bickerstaff

History
General questions

Usually patients present with a combination of symptoms relating to pain, swelling, locking, clicking and giving way; these form the basis of the specific questions asked on taking a history. The diagnostic specificity of each of these symptoms in isolation is poor; rather they are used in combination to guide the examiner to a differential diagnosis. In addition, the presence and degree of each of these symptoms at presentation and how they have changed with the passage of time is important.

It is then important to ascertain the duration of symptoms, exact details of the mechanism of injury and then the general course of events, including response to any treatment already received. It is through this aspect of the history that one obtains a clear picture of the degree of disability suffered by the patient.

Other key questions include occupation, sport and lifestyle.

Specific questions
Pain

The site of pain within the knee is an indication as to the structure damaged but is by no means diagnostic, particularly with traumatic disorders such as meniscal tears. As an example, lateral joint pain from a patellofemoral disorder is frequently mistaken for a lateral meniscal tear. The site of pain following an episode of injury, however, such as a medial collateral ligament (MCL) strain, is a clear indication of the possible structures involved. It is useful to obtain a description of the pain at the time of injury or presentation and

then how the pain has progressed. Of particular importance is whether the pain is constant and whether it occurs at night. For instance, these symptoms are an indication to recommend arthroplasty in assessing a patient with severe degenerative changes. Constant pain may indicate more sinister pathology such as tumour or infection.

It is then important to relate the pain to the level and type of activity, such as whether the symptom appears after a few steps walking or only after running. In addition, questions about the pain related to specific actions such as twisting and turning may indicate a problem with the main weightbearing areas of the knee such as a meniscal tear or chondral defect. Bent-knee activities such as kneeling, crouching or squatting may indicate a patellofemoral problem, although posterior horn tears of the medial meniscus are aggravated by loaded bent-knee activities such as coming up from a squatting position.

The examiner should always be aware of the possibility of referred pain from the hip or lumbar spine, particularly when assessing a patient with degenerative symptoms.

Swelling

Swelling can be outside the joint, such as with a lateral meniscal cyst, or inside the joint, such as with a haemarthrosis. The timing of the swelling is important. Immediate swelling or within a few hours is an indication of haemarthrosis. Gradual swelling indicates effusion.

Generalized swelling may be secondary to a haemarthrosis, which is generally defined as swelling appearing within 4 hours of an injury. The main differential diagnosis of a haemarthrosis is an anterior

Examination Techniques in Orthopaedics, Second Edition, ed. Nick Harris and Fazal Ali. Published by Cambridge University Press. © Cambridge University Press 2014.

cruciate ligament (ACL) rupture, an osteochondral fracture (often associated with a patellar dislocation) or a peripheral meniscal tear. Indeed, if an athlete gives a history of a twisting injury on the sports field followed by swelling within 4 hours, they have a 70–80% chance of having sustained an ACL rupture.[1] The commonest misdiagnosis in this setting is to confuse an ACL rupture with a lateral patellar dislocation. Indeed, rarely, both can occur together.[2] Both occur on the slightly flexed weightbearing knee forced into external rotation. This reinforces the need for a skyline radiograph in the acutely injured knee to identify a possible osteochondral fragment from the patellofemoral joint that occurs in patellar dislocation.

Haemarthroses are painful owing to the degree of tension within the knee. A relatively painless haemarthrosis or diffuse swelling rather than true haemarthrosis should alert the examiner to the possibility of a more extensive ligamentous injury with disruption of the capsule. The examiner can be lulled into thinking that the injury is less severe than is the case.

Locking

Locking can be subdivided into true locking and pseudolocking. True locking is relatively rare. It occurs when an intra-articular structure, loose body or meniscal tear interposes between the femoral condyle and tibial surface. Classically the patient can lose terminal extension but is able to flex the knee (though usually also losing some terminal flexion, which is less noticeable). Loose bodies may also be felt by the patient in the suprapatellar pouch but more commonly in either the medial or lateral gutter. They are classically elusive and, once found, immediately move to another area, hence their eponym of 'joint mouse'.

Pseudolocking is a far more common presentation and usually occurs in patients with anterior knee pain secondary to some form of patellar maltracking. Classically it is associated with marked pain and there is no movement of the knee.

Giving way

There are two types of giving way: true giving way, which is usually associated with some form of ligamentous instability; and a buckling type sensation, which is usually associated with anterior knee pain and the symptom of pseudolocking described above.

An example of true giving way is seen in ACL instability. The patient has no problem running in a straight line but, on planting the foot and twisting with the upper body internally rotating, the knee suddenly collapses quickly.

Instability resulting from chronic medial instability usually presents with difficulty performing cutting movements rather than rotation. Isolated posterior cruciate ligament (PCL) rupture does not usually present with instability unless there is associated posterolateral or posteromedial instability. In these situations the knee again feels unstable with rotatory movements but also on walking downstairs because of the unimpeded anterior displacement of the femur on the tibia.

Buckling of the knee is seen in patients with anterior knee pain and is associated with pain. These patients often report their knee buckling without any rotary movement, usually occurring when walking in a straight line or down stairs. The knee buckling is rarely associated with an effusion.

General examination

Examination of the knee should follow the usual orthopaedic routine of inspection, palpation, movement and ligaments. Specific tests related to the presumed diagnosis should then be addressed; for example, patellofemoral pathology, meniscal tears or other ligaments. One must always remember to use the opposite limb for comparison and, to gain the patient's trust, leave any possible painful tests until the end. A tense patient will make any assessment of subtle instabilities impossible.

The examination should start immediately the patient enters the clinic, to assess their gait, walking aids and general mobility. To assess the patient fully, however, he or she should be undressed from mid thigh.

Inspection

Initial inspection should begin with the **patient standing** to assess overall limb alignment and any shortening.

The **Q angle** (quadriceps angle) has an influence on patellofemoral symptoms by affecting the line of pull of the quadriceps muscle on the patella. It is the angle between a line drawn from the anterior superior iliac spine and the midpoint of the patella with another line drawn from the tibial tubercle through the midpoint of the patella (Figure 9.1a). It averages 15°, with females having a slightly larger angle than males because of the width of the pelvis.

Limb alignment includes any femoral or tibial rotational malalignments which also have a bearing on knee function (Figures 9.1b–e).

Foot position should be assessed for evidence of any abnormalities, such as hyperpronation which again can affect patellofemoral function. It is easier at this stage to assess the posterior aspect of the knee for scars, swellings or bruising. The anterior aspect can be assessed at this stage or later when the patient is supine.

The next step is to **observe the gait pattern**. There should be sufficient room to watch the patient walking both towards and away from the examiner (Figure 9.2a). Important things to observe as the patient walks are the foot progression angle (angle that the foot makes with an imaginary straight line: 10–15° external) and the patellar progression angle (angle that the patella makes with an imaginary straight line: 0°). This would indicate rotational malalignment.

A varus or valgus thrust may also be important signs. Varus thrust may indicate medial compartment osteoarthritis or lateral ligament laxity (Figure 9.2b). A valgus thrust may indicate lateral compartment osteoarthritis or medial ligament laxity.

Next the **patient is sat down** with the legs hanging over the side of the couch (Figure 9.3). Patellar height is best demonstrated here. Ask the patient to extend and flex the knees to feel crepitus and to observe patellar tracking. A J-sign can be observed in some cases. Here the patella moves centrally then subluxes laterally as the knee comes into extension. This is seen in some cases of patellar instability, commonly in tall individuals with generalized laxity.

The **patient is now laid supine** on the examination couch with the head relaxed on a pillow and hands placed on the chest. A patient straining to watch an examination may increase muscle tone, affecting observations such as knee laxity. As well as inspecting the anterior aspect of the knee for scars, swellings or bruising, any quadriceps or calf wasting can be observed and measured from a fixed bony point such as the anterior superior iliac spine (Figure 9.4).

(a)

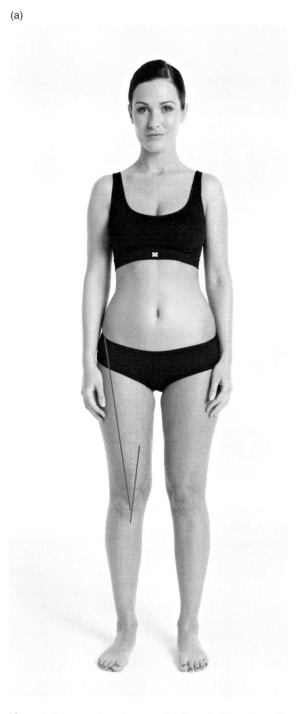

Figure 9.1 Inspect the patient standing from the front, side and back. **a** The Q angle is the angle formed between a line drawn from the anterior superior iliac spine to the midpoint of the patella with a line drawn from the tibial tubercle through the midpoint of the patella. **b** Valgus right knee. **c** Bilateral varus knees. **d** Fixed flexion deformity of the knee. **e** Young patient with miserable malalignment syndrome with both patellae pointing inwards.

(b) (c)

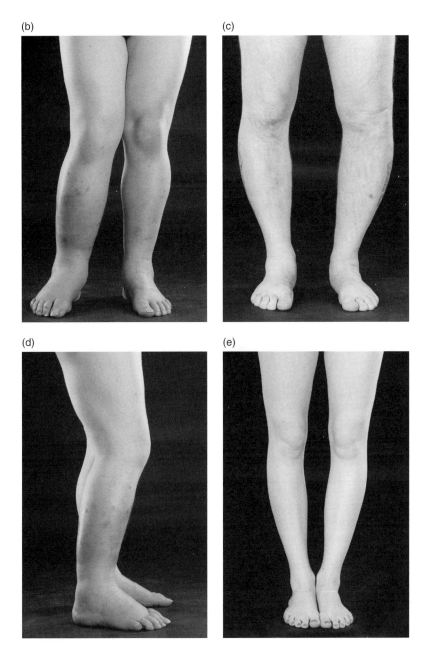

(d) (e)

Figure 9.1 (cont.)

Palpation

There are three basic tests for the presence of an effusion: the ballottment test, the patellar tap test and the wipe (or bulge) test. The **ballottment test** is for a massive effusion and is performed like a fluid thrill test for abdominal ascites. In this test, pressure on one side is transmitted via the fluid to the hand on the other side of the knee. The **patellar tap test** is for moderate effusion (Figure 9.5a). A hand is placed over the suprapatellar pouch and pressed on to occlude this space. The patella is then pressed with the other hand to allow the patella to touch the femoral trochlea. In the presence of a moderate effusion this gives the sensation of a tap. The **wipe/bulge test** is performed for a small effusion (Figure 9.5b). Here the suprapatellar pouch is occluded with one hand. Stroke the lateral gutter and watch the fluid move across to the medial side with a bulge (or vice versa).

(a)

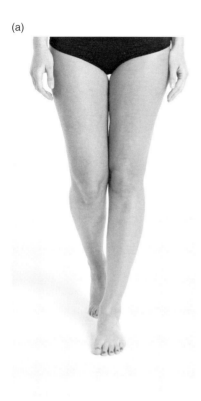

(b)

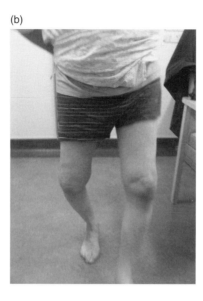

Figure 9.2 a When walking look for rotational abnormalities as well as any lurch. **b** Patient walking with a varus thrust as he weightbears on his right leg.

If there is an appearance of swelling in the knee and yet no effusion, one must consider synovial hypertrophy as seen in conditions such as pigmented villonodular synovitis.[3]

The knee is largely subcutaneous apart from posteriorly and, as such, many structures can be palpated directly. The anatomical location of the tenderness is usually a good indicator of the underlying pathology. This is best done with the knee bent up to 90° with the foot firmly planted on the examination couch in a neutral position (Figure 9.6). The fingers can then be used to palpate along the joint lines, starting with the painless side. Tenderness along the joint line, particularly posteromedially, may indicate a meniscal tear. The borders of the femoral and tibial condyles, the patellar tendon, and medial (MCL) and lateral (LCL) collateral ligaments can also be palpated for tenderness.

The patellar tendon should be palpated in full extension and then tensed at 90° of flexion. In chronic patellar tendinosis, tenderness in the proximal tendon is more noticeable in extension. In flexion the normal superficial fibres cover the damaged deep fibres, resulting in less pain on palpation.

The posterior aspect of the knee should also be palpated to identify soft tissue masses in the popliteal fossa, which may not have been evident on inspection.

Movement

The assessment of movement relates to active and passive movement of the joint. The normal range of passive movement is assessed, comparing both sides and including hyperextension. The range can be noted as degrees of movement. Alternatively, hyperextension can be measured as the distance the heel can be lifted off the examination couch and flexion by the heel to buttock distance. The patient should be asked to actively perform a straight leg raise to assess the integrity of the extensor mechanism and flex the knee as far as possible (Figure 9.7).

Ligament testing

ACL and PCL instability

The first step in assessing ACL or PCL instability involves both knees viewed from the side when flexed to 90° to identify any posterior sag indicating PCL injury. The levels of the tibial tubercles are compared

(Figures 9.8a, b). If posterior sag is not recognized, anterior movement from an abnormally posterior-placed tibia may be misinterpreted as anterior instability.

If there is a positive posterior sag then the **quadriceps active test** can be performed. This test works by contractions of the quadriceps being transmitted to the tibial tubercle via the patella and the patellar tendon. It is performed by fixing the foot and asking the patient to try to extend the leg (Figure 9.8c). If there is a posterior sag the quadriceps will pull the tibia forwards.

In the **anterior and posterior drawer tests** the knees are flexed to 90° and the feet are fixed to the couch. Sitting on the patient's feet has been described; however, this is not usually necessary and can be painful. Both hands are used to grasp the upper tibia, with the thumbs on the tibial tubercles (Figure 9.9). At this angle of flexion the anterior tibial condyles should be anterior to the corresponding femoral condyles. From the neutral position excessive movement forward indicates a positive anterior drawer sign and excessive movement backwards indicates a positive posterior drawer sign. A positive posterior drawer suggests a PCL rupture. A positive anterior drawer suggests an ACL rupture. However, because secondary restraints such as the posterior capsule prevent the tibia coming forward, a positive anterior drawer would suggest not only an injury to the ACL but also to the secondary restraints.

As such if the anterior drawer test is repeated with the foot in external rotation it tests the posteromedial capsule (Slocum test). If the foot is placed in internal rotation it tests the posterolateral capsule.

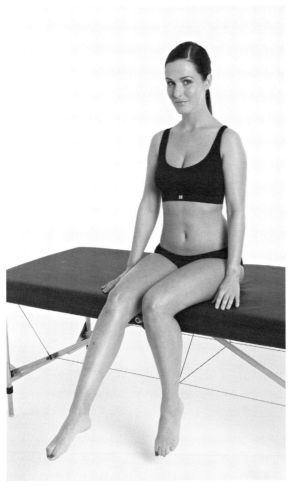

Figure 9.3 Patient sitting with legs hanging freely over side of couch. Assess patellar height, tracking and crepitus.

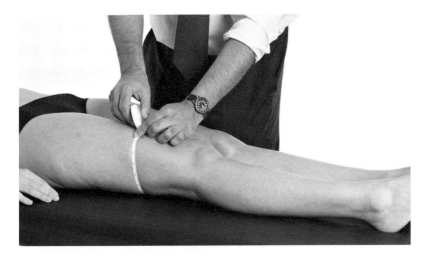

Figure 9.4 Lie the patient comfortably on the couch. Muscle bulk may be assessed by measuring the circumference of the thigh from a fixed point such as the anterior superior iliac spine.

(b)

(a)

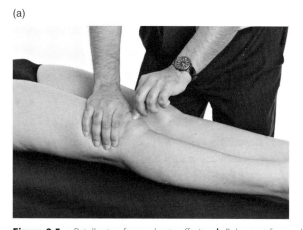

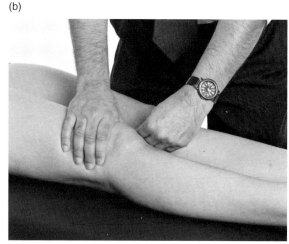

Figure 9.5 a Patellar tap for moderate effusion. **b** Bulge test for small effusion.

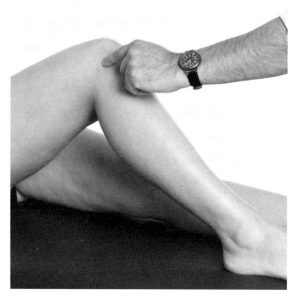

Figure 9.6 Palpation of the knee joint is best done in the flexed knee.

The most reliable test for ACL instability is the **Lachman test**.[4] With a normal sized knee the best technique is to grasp the distal femur with one hand, holding the femur still while flexing the knee to 20°; the other hand then grasps the proximal tibia and displaces the tibia anteriorly (Figure 9.10a). The amount of anterior displacement is then estimated and can be graded. The presence or absence of an endpoint is important to note. Absence of an end-point is indicative of a complete rupture.

In patients with large thighs or examiners with small hands, it is better to fix the femur over the examiner's flexed knee while displacing the tibia with the other hand (Figure 9.10b).[5]

The other classic test for ACL instability is the **pivot shift test**[6], which can be performed a number of different ways, although the basic principle is the same. The pivot shift test recreates the anterolateral subluxation of the tibia on the femur, which results in the giving way sensation experienced by the patient when twisting on a planted foot. The pivot shift test measures the rotational component of ACL function whereas the anterior drawer and Lachman tests measure the anteroposterior stability.

In this test the patient's leg is held in full extension and the lower leg is then internally rotated and a valgus strain applied to the knee via the laterally placed hand. In this position, the tibia is anterolaterally subluxed. The knee is then flexed gently and at about 20° the tibia suddenly reduces; this can be seen in obvious cases and palpated in more subtle cases (Figure 9.11). The degree of instability is increased if the hip is abducted as this decreases tension in the iliotibial band.[7] It is not possible to perform this test with medial instability as the medial pivot is lost. The key to this test is obtaining the patient's confidence as, if performed too forcibly, it can be distressing for the patient. Sometimes, with the leg securely held by the hands around the knee the patient feels more confident, allowing this test to be performed gently and quickly.

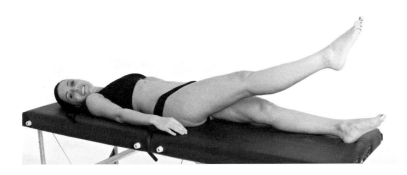

Figure 9.7 Range of movement involves extension and flexion. Here, active straight leg raising demonstrates an intact extensor mechanism.

This test is more commonly performed under anaesthetic rather than in clinics or examinations.

MCL and LCL instability

MCL injuries result in the commonest form of knee instability.

With the leg held above and below the knee it is then placed in full extension. A valgus force is then applied to the knee by pushing the lower leg, held by the elbow and body, against the laterally placed hand. The degree of opening can be assessed but the most important point is whether there is a soft or hard endpoint. If there is no endpoint with the leg in full extension, this signifies a major disruption of the knee with additional damage to the cruciate ligaments and posteromedial capsule which act as secondary stabilizers to valgus

(a)

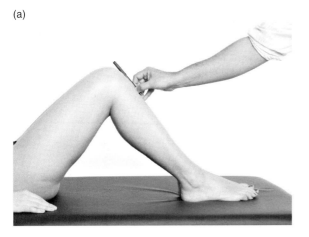

(b)

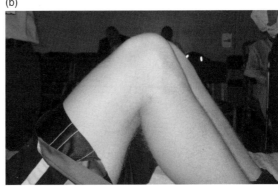

(c)

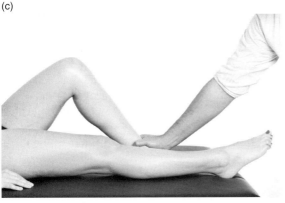

Figure 9.8 a Cruciate ligament testing starts with both knees flexed to 90° and observing the level of the tibial tubercles from the side (posterior sag). **b** A positive posterior sag indicating a ruptured PCL. **c** Quadriceps active test to confirm the posterior sag.

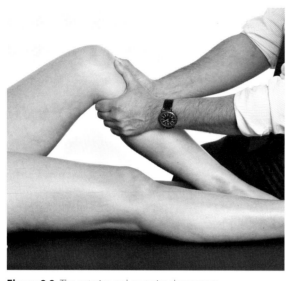

Figure 9.9 The anterior and posterior drawer test.

strain. Some opening with an endpoint may be present with disruption of the deep fibres of the MCL.

The test is then performed in 20–30° of flexion, which relaxes the secondary restraints and allows an assessment of the superficial fibres of the MCL (Figure 9.12a). Again, an assessment is made as to the degree of movement and the presence of an endpoint.

Posteromedial rotatory instability is a major instability involving damage to the posteromedial structures of the knee,[8] principally the posterior oblique ligament. This condition occurs with severe ligament disruptions, usually affecting the PCL. As well as medial opening in extension, the posterior subluxation of the medial tibial plateau off the femur can be demonstrated by performing a valgus stress.

LCL instability in isolation is less common than MCL isolation, and is often associated with posterolateral instability, which will be described in the next

(a)

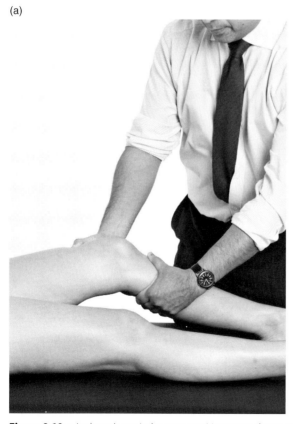

(b)

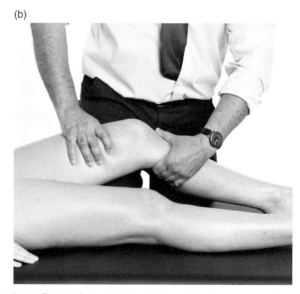

Figure 9.10 a Lachman's test is the most sensitive test to detect an ACL insufficiency. **b** In patients with large thighs this may be better performed in the position shown here with the examiner's thigh under the patient's thigh.

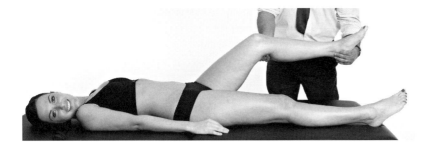

Figure 9.11 The pivot shift test.

(b)

(a)

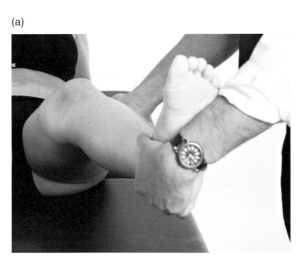

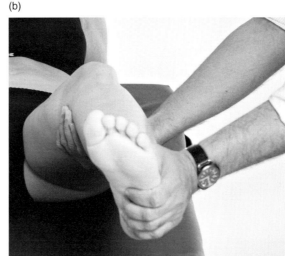

Figure 9.12 Testing collateral ligaments. **a** MCL and **b** LCL.

section. Essentially, however, the test is the same as for the MCL (Figure 9.12b). There is greater normal laxity in the lateral structures and care should be taken to compare movement with the uninjured knee.

Further tests

Posterolateral rotatory instability

Posterolateral corner (PLC) injuries can be isolated but are more commonly associated with PCL and ACL injuries.

There are many tests described to diagnose posterolateral instability. Some of the more common ones will be described here. The key to the clinical examination features is increased external rotation. These patients may also walk with a pronounced varus/lateral thrust.

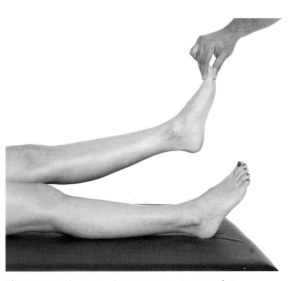

Figure 9.13 The external rotation recurvatum test for posterolateral corner injuries.

(b)

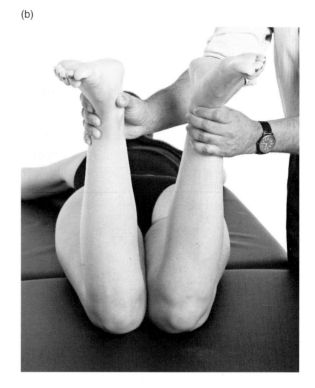

(a)

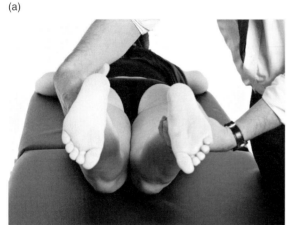

(c)

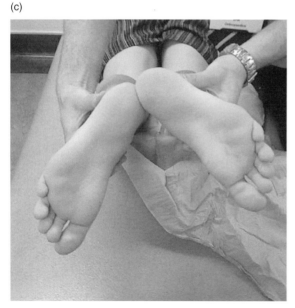

Figure 9.14 The dial test. The tibia is externally rotated at **a** 30° and **b** 90° of flexion. **c** Patient with positive dial test, which indicates a posterolateral corner injury.

The **external rotation recurvatum test** involves lifting both legs off the couch by grasping the great toes (Figure 9.13). A positive result is when the knee goes into varus and hyperextension (recurvatum) and externally rotates.

The **posterolateral drawer sign** is demonstrated by performing the posterior drawer test in neutral alignment, with the tibia internally rotated and then with the tibia externally rotated. An increase in magnitude of the posterior drawer in external rotation indicates a PLC injury.[9]

The **dial test** is passive external rotation of the tibia (relative to the femur), with the knee at 30° and 90° of flexion (Figures 9.14a, b). This is best performed with the patient prone. The knees are kept together to prevent rotation at the hips. It is also best to control the rotation of the tibia by grasping above the ankles. The feet indicate the angle of rotation from neutral. In the rare case of isolated PLC injury, increased external rotation is noted at 30° but this is less so at 90°. When combined PCL and PLC injuries are present, increased external rotation is noted in both positions (Figure 9.14c).[10]

Limb alignment and gait pattern must be observed to ensure that there is no lateral thrust on walking (which is seen in chronic posterolateral rotatory instability), usually associated with PCL injury but also seen in ACL injury. If this is not recognized, the ligament reconstructions may fail in the absence of a corrective osteotomy.

PLC injuries are major events and in the acute setting particular care must be taken to ensure that there is no neurovascular injury, in particular to the common peroneal nerve.

Meniscal pathology

The **Apley grind test** is historical and involves forcing the tibiofemoral surfaces together to catch the meniscus. In this test the patient is prone with the knee flexed to 90° and the examiner pushes downwards on the foot and rotates the leg.

McMurray's test was to recreate displacement of a meniscal tear; this is painful and probably not in the patient's best interests. A modification of this is a compression test to produce discomfort along the joint line, which may indicate pathology in the medial or lateral compartment.[11] The patient is supine with the knee flexed. The examiner places one hand on the top of the knee with the fingers and thumbs positioned to palpate the joint line, and the other hand under the heel (Figure 9.15). The examiner can then compress the joint by pushing down on the top hand while the lower hand controls flexion and can also rotate the leg, thereby stressing each compartment in varying degrees of flexion. This test is most specific for a tear of the posterior horn of the medial meniscus.

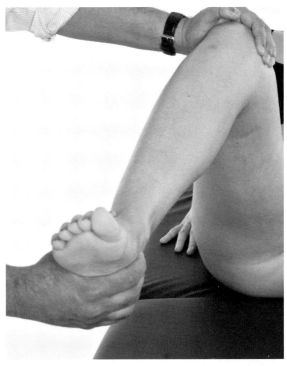

Figure 9.15 McMurray's test is a provocative test for meniscal pathology.

Another, less specific, test is to ask the patient to squat fully, and, if possible, duck walk (Childress' test). This action compresses the posterior horns of the menisci but can also cause patellofemoral pain.

Diagnosis is made from the history and tenderness along the joint line. The absence of positive signs does not definitely exclude a meniscal tear but other investigations such as an MRI scan should be undertaken.

Patellofemoral pathology

The commonest patellofemoral pathologies include maltracking, which manifests in pain, subluxation or frank dislocation and osteoarthritis.

An assessment of the overall alignment of the leg, including rotational malalignment and abnormal foot position, has already been mentioned.

An assessment should then be made of lateral retinacular tightness, which is found with patellar tilting such as is seen in excessive lateral pressure syndrome. To do this the patella should

(a)

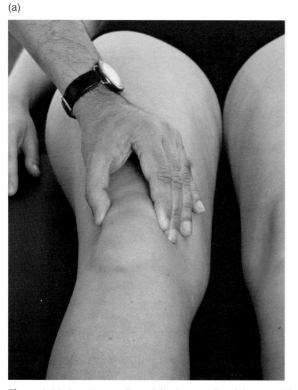

(b)

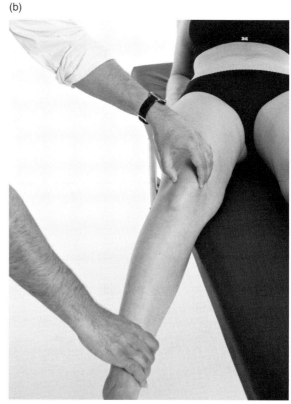

Figure 9.16 Assessing patellar stability by **a** patellar glide test and **b** patellar apprehension test.

be just engaged in the femoral trochlea. In the **patellar glide test** the knee is flexed slightly and the patella is moved maximally medially and laterally (Figure 9.16a). If one imagines the patella split into quadrants, the patella should be able to move at least one quadrant medially; any less indicates lateral retinacular tightness. The medial retinaculum is naturally more lax, but movement of greater than two quadrants laterally indicates laxity in the medial retinaculum, which one may see in recurrent patellar dislocation. With the patella held in this lateral position, the knee is now flexed and the patient's reaction observed (Figure 9.16b). A positive **patellar apprehension test** is seen when the patient resists further flexion for fear of the patella dislocating.

Clarke's test is used to demonstrate patellofemoral pathology such as chondromalacia and patellofemoral arthritis. In performing this test put a hand over the suprapatellar pouch with gentle pressure on the superior pole of the patella

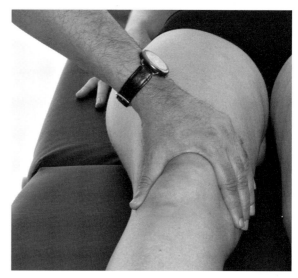

Figure 9.17 Clarke's test for patellofemoral problems.

(Figure 9.17). Ask the patient to contract the quadriceps or to attempt a straight leg raise. Pain in the patellofemoral joint indicates that pathology is present.

Summary

Summary of knee examination

Step 1
Stand the patient and look

Step 2
Walk the patient

Step 3
Sit the patient down

- Assess patellar height, tracking and crepitus

Step 4
Lie the patient down

- Look (quantify quadriceps wasting)
- Feel effusion or tenderness
- Move

Step 5
Assess ligaments:

- Cruciates
- Collaterals

Step 6
Further tests based on findings above:

a. Meniscal
b. Ligamentous
c. Patellofemoral.

Stand and look

On standing the patient inspect from the front, side, both laterally and medially and the popliteal fossa at the back. Note any scars, wasting, swelling or deformity. It is also important to comment on the Q angle whilst looking from the front and also the rotational profile.

Walk

Comment particularly on any obvious varus or valgus lurch. Also note the foot and patellar progression angles.

Sit

Whilst the patient is sitting look at the patellar height. Ask the patient to extend his or her knee, in particular looking at the patellar tracking and the J-sign, which may be present in ligamentously lax patients with patellar instability. Feel for crepitus.

Lie patient down

Look, feel, move then test the ligaments

Look — Especially at the quadriceps and quantify quadriceps wasting by measuring from a fixed point; for example, the anterior superior iliac spine.

Feel — Effusion:

- Wipe or bulge test for mild effusion
- Patellar tap for moderate effusion
- Ballottment test for significant effusion.

Continue feeling by resting hands over knee and palpating the popliteal fossa, joint line, tibial tubercle, patellar tendon and medial and lateral collateral ligaments in turn.

Move — Firstly assess extension by asking the patient to perform a straight leg raise; then lift both heels in the hands and assess any degree of recurvatum. Flexion is assessed first actively and then passively, comparing both knees.

Ligaments

Cruciate ligaments — Flex both knees to 90° with heels together. Look from the side and look for a posterior sag. If there is a sag then perform the quadriceps active test. In this test the foot is fixed and the patient is asked to extend the leg. In the presence of a posterior sag the tibia will be pulled forward to a neutral position by the contraction of the quadriceps muscle.

Next, perform the anterior and posterior draw tests.

Follow this with Lachman's test with the knee flexed to 20–30°.

Note that the pivot shift test is not usually recommended for the exam as this test is most commonly and reliably performed in the anaesthetic room as it can be quite painful.

Collateral ligaments — Test the MCL and the LCL in extension and then in 30° of flexion.

Further tests

The above sequence is carried out in all cases of knee examination. After testing the ligaments, proceed in one of **three** directions depending on the previous findings:

1. If there is the likelihood of meniscal pathology, then meniscal provocative tests may be performed.
2. If there is ligamentous pathology, then assessment of the PLC should be carried out. The most common test for this is the dial test.
3. If the findings indicate patellofemoral pathology, then other patellofemoral tests can be carried out such as the patellar glide test, patellar apprehension test and Clarke's test.

References

1   Maffuli N, Binfield PM, King JB, Good CJ. Acute haemarthrosis of the knee in athletes. A prospective study of 106 cases. *J Bone Joint Surg (Br)* 1993;**75**:945–949.

2   Simonian PT, Fealy S, Hidaka C, O'Brien SJ, Warren RF. Anterior cruciate ligament injury and patella dislocation: a report of nine cases. *Arthroscopy* 1998;**14**: 80–84.

3   Flandrey F, Hughston JC, McCann SB, Kurtz DM. Diagnostic features of diffuse pigmented villonodular synovitis of the knee. *Clin Orthop* 1994;**298**:212–220.

4   Torg JS, Conrad W, Kalen V. Clinical diagnosis of anterior cruciate ligament instability in athletes. *Am J Sports Med* 1976; **4**:84–93.

5   Draper DO, Schulthies SS. Examiner proficiency in performing the anterior draw and Lachman tests. *J Orthop Sports Phys Ther* 1995;**22**:263–266.

6   Galway HR, MacIntosh DL. The lateral pivot shift: a symptom and sign of anterior cruciate ligament instability. *Clin Orthop* 1980;**147**:45–50.

7   Bach BR Jr, Warren RF, Wickiewicz TL. The pivot shift phenomenon: results and a description of a modified clinical test for anterior cruciate ligament instability. *Am J Sports Med* 1988;**16**:571–576.

8   Nielsen S, Rasmusson O, Oveson J, Andersen K. Rotatory instability of cadaver knees after transection of collateral ligaments and capsule. *Arch Orthop Trauma Surg* 1984;**103**:165–169.

9   Reider B. *The Orthopaedic Physical Exam*, 2nd edition. Philadelphia: Elsevier Saunders, 2005.

10 Bae JH, Choi IC, Suh SW *et al.* Evaluation of the reliability of the dial test for posterolateral rotator instability: a cadaveric study using an isotonic rotation machine. *Arthroscopy* 2008;**24**:593–598.

11 Solomon L, Warwick D, Nayagam S. *Apley's System of Orthopaedics and Fractures*, 8th edition. London: Edward Arnold, 2001.

Examination of the foot and ankle

Nick Harris and Tom Smith

History

General

Details of age, sex, occupation and problems with shoewear must always be elicited from patients with foot and ankle problems. Pain, swelling, stiffness, deformity, instability and paraesthesiae are the usual complaints. Their effects on gait, leisure and employment activities must be clearly established.

Many systemic conditions affect the foot. This is usually bilateral. A high index of suspicion must be maintained by clinicians managing foot and ankle disorders. Diabetes, rheumatoid arthritis, seronegative arthropathies, endocrinopathies, gout, pseudogout and vasculitic conditions all directly affect the foot and will influence management strategies. Swelling of the foot and ankle might reflect cardiac, hepatic and renal disease.

Unilateral swelling might be the result of secondary obstruction of the lymphatics resulting from pelvic malignancy, especially in women over the age of 50. Painless unilateral swelling of the foot or ankle may be the result of a Charcot joint in a patient with diabetic peripheral neuropathy.

Lesions of the lumbosacral spine, such as a prolapsed intervertebral disc, spina bifida and spinal stenosis, may also affect the foot, and any history of spinal abnormality must be sought.

Specific

The most important complaint in ankle and foot pathology is pain. Pain referral from primary foot pathology is rare except in entrapment neuropathies. Localization to a specific area therefore narrows the diagnosis significantly.

Ankle pain is often felt anteriorly, especially in degenerative disease with impingement. Rheumatoid involvement in the ankle is less common than in the other joints of the foot and is usually manifest as a tenosynovitis.

Ankle instability presents in two ways, either recurrent sprains or a feeling of looseness when walking on uneven ground or wearing high-heeled shoes. Pain is an uncommon feature unless there is an associated talar lesion. Tarsal coalition may present with ankle instability.

Pain in the subtalar joint is often localized below and behind the malleoli and also in the sinus tarsi. Vanio[1] stated that 60–70% of patients with rheumatoid arthritis will have involvement of the subtalar and midtarsal joints. The resulting deformity is one of valgus, with patients complaining that the foot is gradually 'going over'. Tibialis posterior tenosynovitis may exacerbate this.

Heel pain may be localized to either side of the calcaneus, especially in conditions such as insufficiency fractures of the calcaneus and Paget's disease. Pain at the insertion of the Achilles' tendon and plantar fascia is associated with systemic conditions such as gout, pseudogout and seronegative arthropathies, especially when bilateral. Unilateral plantar fasciitis and Achilles' tendonitis usually result from biomechanical and environmental factors, which result in microtears and inflammation. Burning pain anterior to the medial calcaneal tuberosity on the plantar aspect of the foot, which is worse with the first few steps in the morning, is typical of plantar fasciitis. The presence of a plantar heel spur on X-ray neither confirms nor refutes the existence of plantar fasciitis. Pain located to the insertion of the Achilles' tendon made worse with resisted plantarflexion activities is typical of Achilles' tendonitis.

Examination Techniques in Orthopaedics, Second Edition, ed. Nick Harris and Fazal Ali. Published by Cambridge University Press. © Cambridge University Press 2014.

Table 10.1 Metatarsalgia

Callosity	No callosity	
	Neuritic symptoms	No neuritic symptoms
Hallux valgus	Morton's neuroma	MTP instability
Bunionette	Tarsal tunnel syndrome	MTP capsulitis
Claw, hammer, mallet toe	PID	Stress fracture
IPK		

IPK, intractable plantar keratosis; PID, prolapsed intervertebral disc.

Table 10.2 Differential diagnosis of acquired cavovarus foot

Neuromuscular	Cerebral palsy Spinal dysraphism Spinal cord tumour Poliomyelitis Hereditary motor and sensory neuropathy (Charcot–Marie–Tooth disease) Muscular dystrophy
Structural	Trauma

Pain and swelling posterior to the medial malleolus along the course of the posterior tibial tendon often reflects posterior tibial tendonitis. Any loss of the normal medial arch, as in acquired pes planus, might also suggest attenuation or rupture of the posterior tibial tendon.

Posteromedial pain might also represent flexor hallucis longus (FHL) tendonitis. Pain of this origin is typically made worse by movement of the hallux. In severe cases, triggering of the hallux can occur resulting from FHL tendon stenosis between the medial and lateral tubercles of the talus. Lateral ankle pain can be caused by peroneal tendonitis and subluxation.

Midfoot pain is less common than hindfoot and forefoot pain. Post-traumatic, degenerative and inflammatory arthritic conditions can all lead to midfoot pain. In the diabetic patient swelling of the midfoot with or without pain is typical of Charcot neuroarthropathy of the midtarsal joint if there is no evidence of infection. Navicular stress fractures are also a cause of midfoot pain, especially in athletes.

Forefoot pain or metatarsalgia has many causes. It is simplified by initially establishing whether the patient has an associated callosity or not and, secondly, whether the patient has neuritic symptoms.[2] Table 10.1 outlines a simple algorithm to help in diagnosis. Patients with hallux valgus and lesser toe deformities complain of difficulties with shoewear and unsightliness, as well as pain.

Symmetrical clawing of the lesser toes and deformity of the hallux is typical of the rheumatoid forefoot. The synovitis causes extension of the metatarsophalangeal (MTP) joints, with subsequent rupture of the volar plate leading to clawing of the toes. The clawed toes pull the plantar fat pad distally and expose the metatarsal heads. Patients describe a feeling of 'walking on pebbles'.

Intractable plantar keratosis (IPK) usually occurs under the second or third metatarsals and is the result of either a transfer lesion because of medial column insufficiency (for example, such as in hallux valgus) or because of problems with the ray itself, such as metatarsal overlength. Patients complain of well localized plantar pain directly beneath the metatarsal head on weightbearing.

Nerve compression or irritation can occur at many levels. An accurate history will help to localize the pathology. Local lesions can cause narrowing of the tarsal tunnel such as a ganglion, schwannoma or lipoma. Systemic conditions such as myxoedema must not be forgotten as a cause of nerve compression. Patients with tarsal tunnel syndrome complain of vague diffuse burning pain and tingling over the plantar aspect of the foot which is often worse with exercise. Occasionally, patients complain of pain radiating up the medial aspect of the leg (Valleix phenomenon).

In contrast, patients with a Morton's neuroma complain of a burning plantar pain well localized between the metatarsal heads. The pain often radiates to the toes of the involved interspace, usually the third and fourth. Atypical neuritic symptoms should alert the physician to more proximal lesions such as a prolapsed intervertebral disc and mononeuritis of diabetes.

Acquired foot deformity in the adult typically presents with pain associated with overloading. The acquired cavovarus foot has either a neuromuscular or traumatic aetiology (Table 10.2). Patients with a cavovarus deformity often complain of pain under the metatarsal heads together with lateral instability. They also complain of uneven shoewear in the early stages. The acquired flat foot deformity in the adult often results from posterior tibial tendon dysfunction, rheumatoid disease, trauma, infection or tumour (classically osteoid osteoma). Pain is often felt medially over the prominent talar head and laterally resulting from impingement of the lateral talar process in the angle of Gissane. Tarsal coalition usually presents in childhood but can present in adults with a fixed planus deformity and ankle instability.

General examination

Inspection

The patient is first examined standing. Many foot and ankle deformities have a neurological basis, therefore from behind the first area to inspect is the lumbar spine for signs suggestive of spinal dysraphism such as a hairy patch, naevus, lipoma, dimple or sinus (Figure 10.1a).

Patients with generalized hyperlaxity frequently have foot problems such as flat feet. Beighton's scoring (see Chapter 1) may confirm this.

(a)

(b)

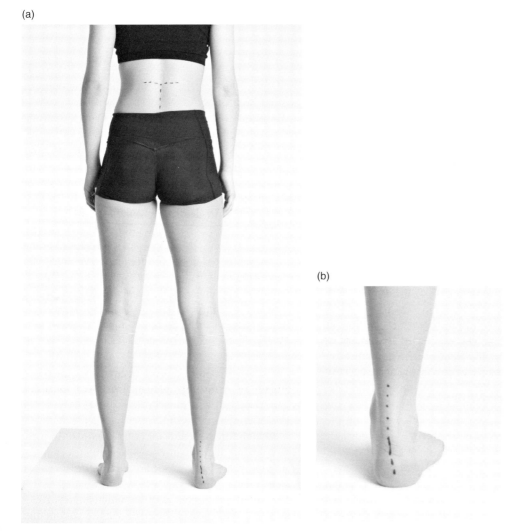

Figure 10.1 a Stand the patient and look from the front, sides and back. Pay particular attention to any deformity, the arches and the hindfoot. Remember to look at the spine. **b** The tibiocalcaneal angle – usually 5° of valgus.

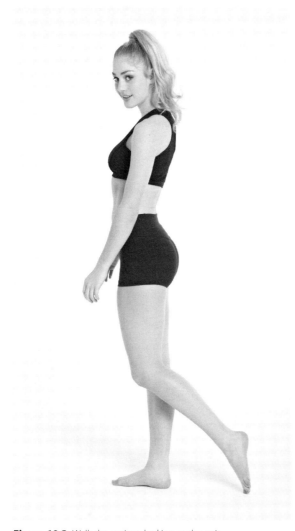

Figure 10.2 Walk the patient, looking at the gait.

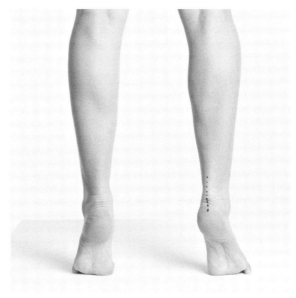

Figure 10.3 Ask the patient to tip toe, observing the arches.

The position of the heel in relation to the floor is best assessed from the back, as is any asymmetry of the calves. Swelling of the Achilles' tendon or posteromedial or posterolateral aspects of the ankle are also best assessed from behind. In this position the relationship between the long axis of the tibia and the long axis of the os calcis should be commented on. This represents the tibiocalcaneal angle and is usually 5° of valgus (Figure 10.1b).

From behind the patient it is also possible to comment on the amount of the forefoot visible. This has important implications in patients with posterior tibial tendon disruption; for example, the 'too-many-toes sign'. Normally about one and a half toes are visible when looking from behind. More than this, or

asymmetry between the two sides, indicates that the arch has dropped.

From the front the examiner should start with the ankle, commenting on any swelling that might represent synovitis, an effusion or osteophytes. Moving anteriorly, the examiner then comments on the medial longitudinal arch. The arch may be flatter than expected (planus) or higher than expected (cavus). There may also be deformity of the midfoot.

The forefoot can have many different deformities in the same foot. It is important to describe the deformities in a logical fashion, starting with the hallux and moving laterally. Skin and nail changes must be sought, especially in diabetic patients (where ulceration is common) and patients with psoriasis (where pitting of the nails can be found).

Walking the patient may be regarded as part of inspection (Figure 10.2). Walking can reveal disability, pain or stiffness. A patient with an arthritic ankle will have difficulty moving through the second rocker of gait. A patient with an arthritic first MTP joint will have difficulty with toe-off.

The standing patient is asked to **rise onto tip toes**. This confirms that the gastrosoleus complex is functioning. If both heels adopt a varus position during this manoeuvre this suggests that both tibialis posterior tendons are functioning as well (Figure 10.3). Doing this is especially important if the patient has a pes planus. Here a single-leg tip toe test can be performed. If the patient has a pes cavus, then

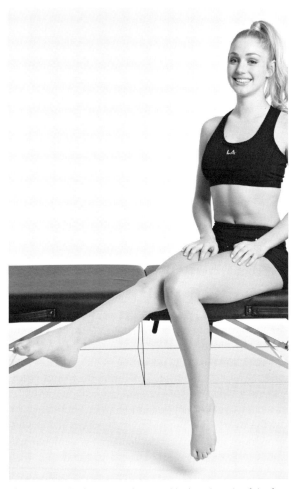

Figure 10.4 Sit the patient down and look at the sole of the foot and between the toes.

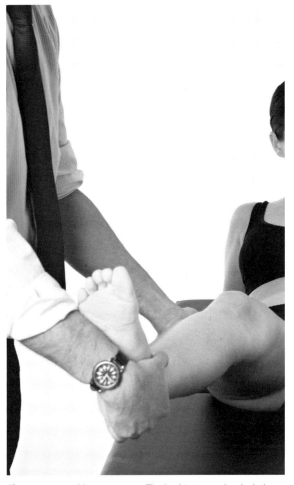

Figure 10.5 Ankle movements. The heel is inverted to lock the subtalar joint and the forefoot is supinated slightly by resting it on the forearm.

consider performing a Coleman block test at this stage. Both of these tests are described below.

Finally, the **plantar aspect of the foot** and between the toes must be inspected for evidence of plantar keratoses or ulcers. Diabetic ulcers are typically found under the first metatarsal head, the pulp of the hallux and beneath the second and third metatarsal heads. The patient may need to be seated to inspect the plantar aspect (Figure 10.4). Do not forget to look for shoes and walking aids, as these will give an indication of any pressure points in the foot and any degree of disability.

Movement

Active and passive **ankle movement** is assessed with the patient seated, both with the knee flexed and extended. Ideally it is best to have the legs hanging over the side of the couch. The usual range of ankle movement is 20° of dorsiflexion and 40° of plantar-flexion. An ankle that cannot plantarflex to neutral is described as being in *calcaneus*.

Passive movement must be assessed with the fore-foot in supination to exclude dorsiflexion at Chopart's and the midtarsal joints. Inversion of the heel to lock the subtalar joint will further ensure that the passive movement is isolated to the ankle joint. To examine, put one hand on the heel and invert it to lock the subtalar joint. Use the same forearm to support the foot (Figure 10.5). The other hand supports the tibia. Dorsiflex the ankle by lifting the forearm under the foot. Plantarflex by bringing it downwards. Alterna-tively, the heel can be inverted to lock the subtalar joint and the forefoot supinated to lock the midfoot.

Causes of reduced ankle dorsiflexion include:

- Primary problems within the joint such as ankle arthritis
- Obstruction from the front either by soft tissue or osteophytes (impingement), usually seen in footballers, ballet dancers and other sports' persons
- Contracture or tightness of the gastrocnemius (assessed by Silfverskiöld's test, described below)
- Scarring of the tibiofibular syndesmosis. The widest part of the talus is anterior, therefore to achieve full dorsiflexion the syndesmosis has to separate slightly. If it is damaged or scarred (for example, following ankle sprains or fractures), this separation does not occur and the dorsiflexion is reduced.

Subtalar movement can be assessed with the foot hanging over the side of the couch or can be examined with the patient prone. Giannestras[3] stated that in the plantigrade position there is only 5° of valgus and 5° of varus movement in the subtalar joint. To examine the subtalar joint, hold the calcaneus with one hand and the talar head/neck with the thumb and index finger of the other hand. Apply a varus and valgus stress with the hand that is holding the calcaneus and at the same time feel for movement of the talus with the other hand. Holding the talus isolates subtalar from ankle motion (Figure 10.6).

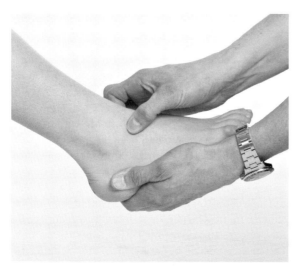

Figure 10.6 Subtalar movements. The talus is felt between the index finger and thumb of one hand. The other hand grasps the patient's heel and inverts/everts it.

Whilst in this position it is possible to assess the relationship of the forefoot to the hindfoot. With the heel aligned with the long axis of the leg, the thumb of the examiner's hand grasping the heel is placed over the talonavicular joint. With the other hand the forefoot is then repeatedly manipulated until it is felt that the talar head is covered by the navicular. This is called the neutral position and in this position the relationship of the forefoot to the hindfoot can be commented upon. The forefoot can adopt one of three positions related to the hindfoot: pronated, supinated or neutral (see below). This manoeuvre is of particular value when constructing orthoses, although it is not commonly performed by most orthopaedic surgeons.

Inversion and eversion are assessed with the foot in a relaxed position of slight plantarflexion to assess inversion, and a neutral position to assess eversion, remembering that these movements reflect movement not just at the subtalar joint but also at Chopart's and the midtarsal joints (Figure 10.7). Whilst performing these movements passively, it is possible to assess whether movement is occurring at the subtalar joint or elsewhere in the foot. The amount of inversion is generally twice that of eversion, approximately 20° of inversion and 10° of eversion.

By fixing the hindfoot, the amount of passive pronation and supination occurring at Chopart's and the midtarsal joints can be assessed and their contribution to overall inversion and eversion can then be calculated. Similarly, by fixing the hindfoot (holding the calcaneum in neutral position with one hand), **abduction and adduction** of the midtarsal joints can be assessed. This movement is minimal (about 5°). Whilst examining the midfoot, pay particular attention to the mobility of the **first tarsometatarsal** joint, which may be a contributing factor in hallux valgus and may need to be addressed by a Lapidus fusion. To assess this joint, use one hand to fix the tarsal bones and the other to grasp the first metatarsal and to move it in a dorsal and plantar direction.

Active and passive **movement of the hallux** is then assessed. The usual range is 80° of dorsiflexion and 40° of plantarflexion relative to the long axis of the first metatarsal. In hallux rigidus, active and passive movement will be restricted and painful. During passive movement it is often easy to demonstrate impingement between the base of the proximal phalanx and the prominent cheilus on the dorsal aspect of

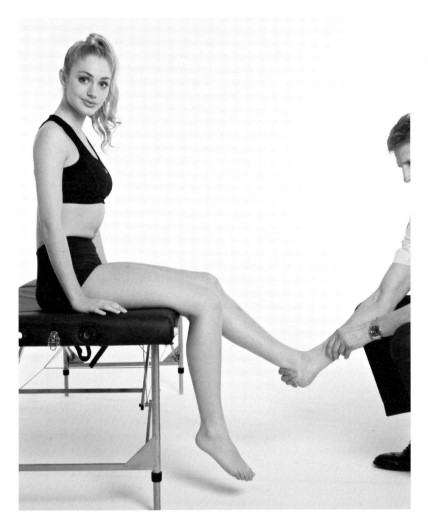

Figure 10.7 Inversion is a combined movement of subtalar joint and midfoot, and is best assessed with the ankle slightly plantarflexed.

the neck of the first metatarsal (Figure 10.8). A **grind test** has been described to support a diagnosis of hallux rigidus. The great toe is grasped, loaded and then rotated in the coronal plane. This reproduces the patient's symptoms if there is complete joint involvement rather than isolated impingement.

Palpation

This must again follow a systematic approach, starting with the ankle and moving distally. It is important to know the anatomy of the underlying structures (Figure 10.9). *Palpation may reveal an area of tenderness that may make the examiner suspicious of a particular diagnosis. It is useful at this point of the clinical examination to perform a special test that may help to confirm the diagnosis.*

Palpation is not complete unless a neurovascular assessment is performed (Figure 10.10).

Medially, the examiner assesses the ankle for swelling or tenderness that might reflect synovitis or rupture of the posterior tibial tendon, irritation or compression of the posterior tibial nerve or snapping of the flexor hallucis longus.

Moving anteriorly in a clockwise fashion, ankle synovitis or an effusion can be felt in the notch of Harty, which is the space medial to the tibialis anterior. Crepitus might also be felt here with passive movement.

Moving laterally, the tibialis anterior, long extensors and peroneus tertius can be palpated. As the examiner moves further lateral the anterolateral aspect of the ankle joint can be palpated. Again, synovitis, an effusion and crepitus can be detected here.

Moving posteriorly the examiner can palpate the peroneal tendons. The calcaneofibular ligament runs deep to the peroneal tendons, creating an angle of approximately 100° with the anterior talofibular ligament. Tenderness in this region may reflect injury to the peroneal tendons, the superior peroneal retinaculum or the calcaneofibular ligament.

Continuing in a clockwise direction the examiner then moves onto the Achilles' tendon. Tenderness, thickening and nodules can be detected as well as any bony swelling such as in a Haglund's deformity. To distinguish between thickenings of the tendon or tendon sheath, passive dorsiflexion and plantar flexion are performed. A thickening of the tendon will move with movement of the tendon whilst a thickening of the sheath will remain fixed.

Having palpated the ankle, the examiner then moves more distally. The calcaneus is the site of origin of the plantar fascia from the anteromedial tuberosity. Tenderness here is indicative of plantar fasciitis. The plantar fascia should also be palpated for plantar fibromatoses. Side-to-side compression of the calcaneus is helpful in identifying patients with structural abnormalities of the heel; for example, stress fractures.

Maximally dorsiflexing the great toe tenses the plantar fascia and may provoke further discomfort. This manoeuvre also recreates the medial longitudinal arch in a patient with a mobile pes planus deformity, the so-called 'windlass effect' (Figure 10.13).

Moving distally, the examiner then palpates Chopart's joint (talonavicular and calcaneocuboid) for evidence of tenderness and/or crepitus. Between the two joints is the sinus tarsi, and tenderness here is often suggestive of irritation of the subtalar joint. The midtarsal joints should be assessed in a similar way.

Moving on to the forefoot, the examiner starts with the hallux. Tenderness and swelling dorsally at the level of the MTP joint is suggestive of a cheilus associated with hallux rigidus. Tenderness and swelling along the shaft of a metatarsal, especially the second, might reflect a stress fracture.

Tenderness and swelling of a lesser MTP joint might reflect a synovitis, such as that associated with Freiberg's disease, which typically affects the second MTP head. Isolated MTP joint synovitis can be detected by passively plantarflexing the toes. This manoeuvre is painful in the presence of synovitis. Swelling and tenderness of all the MTP joints is typical of rheumatoid or psoriatic arthritis. In this case

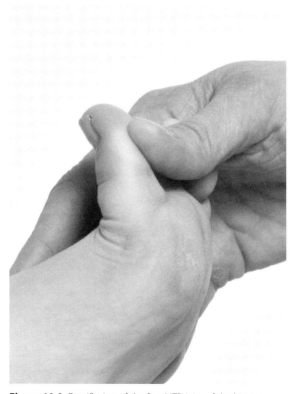

Figure 10.8 Dorsiflexion of the first MTP joint of the big toe.

Thumb pressure applied over the anterolateral gutter with the foot in plantarflexion will push any hypertrophic synovium into the joint, causing pain. If the foot is then moved into dorsiflexion the pain intensifies, which is positive for synovial impingement. This is the **anterolateral impingement test** (Figure 10.11).[4]

From this position the examiner can move superiorly over the inferior tibiofibular syndesmosis. Tenderness here may reflect injury to this structure. A further test to support this is the **squeeze test** where the examiner squeezes the calf at mid calf level, compressing the fibula and tibia in the coronal plane[5] (Figure 10.12). External rotation of the foot with the leg stabilized anteriorly is also a provocative test for syndesmosis injuries.

Moving distal to the joint line the examiner can palpate the anterior talofibular ligament, which runs at an angle of approximately 70° to the long axis of the fibula from the anterodistal aspect of the fibula to the talus. Further anteriorly the sinus tarsi can be palpated. Tenderness here may reflect irritation of the subtalar joint.

(a)

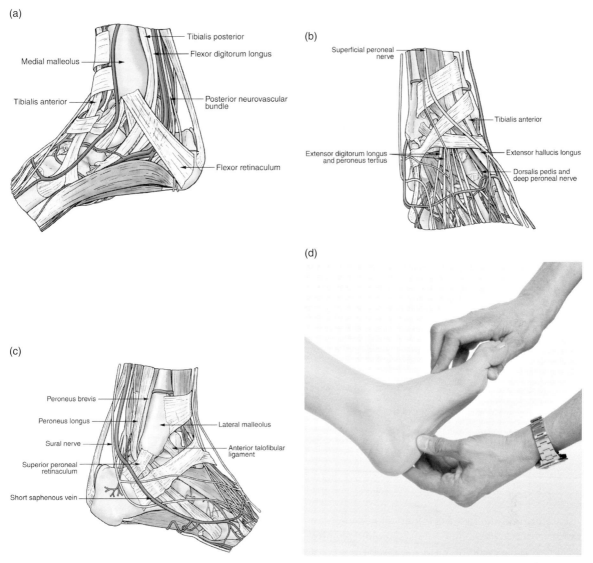

Tibialis posterior

Flexor digitorum longus

Medial malleolus

Tibialis anterior

Posterior neurovascular bundle

Flexor retinaculum

(b)

Superficial peroneal nerve

Tibialis anterior

Extensor digitorum longus and peroneus tertius

Extensor hallucis longus

Dorsalis pedis and deep peroneal nerve

(d)

(c)

Peroneus brevis

Peroneus longus

Sural nerve

Superior peroneal retinaculum

Short saphenous vein

Lateral malleolus

Anterior talofibular ligament

Figure 10.9 Palpation of the foot and ankle systematically. Area of tenderness gives an idea based on the underlying anatomical structures. **a** The anatomy of the medial aspect of the ankle. **b** The anatomy of the anterior aspect of the ankle. **c** The anatomy of the lateral aspect of the ankle. **d** The site of maximum tenderness in patients with plantar fasciitis.

there may be evidence of the 'daylight sign'. Because of the synovitis the toes are pushed apart, so daylight can be seen between each. The 'squeeze test' reinforces this. The toes are squeezed in a medial–lateral direction, which provokes discomfort if a synovitis is present.

Palpation of the plantar aspect of the forefoot attempts to identify specific areas of tenderness, often related to plantar keratoses beneath prominent metatarsal heads.

Tenderness between the metatarsal heads, especially in the third web space and if associated with burning pain and paraesthesiae radiating to the toes, is typical of a Morton's neuroma. Reproduction of the pain when squeezing the toes in a mediolateral direction and the production of a click by applying dorsally directed pressure from beneath the affected web space further support the diagnosis and is described as Mulder's sign (Figure 10.14).[6]

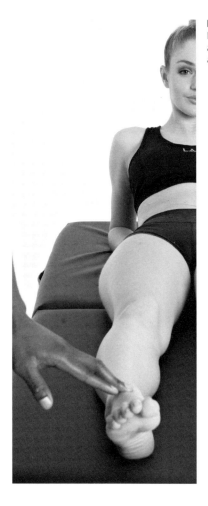

Figure 10.10 Palpation ends with a neurovascular assessment.

Pain beneath the first MTP joint should alert the examiner to the possibility of a sesamoiditis, which can either be the result of a degenerative process or a stress fracture.

Special tests
Coleman block test

This is used in the cavovarus foot. Plantarflexion of the first ray is the result of sparing of the peroneus longus. To move the lateral four metatarsals in to a plantigrade position, the heel must move into varus. The examiner must determine whether the hindfoot varus is fixed or mobile. The Coleman block test[7] is used to distinguish between the two. A block is placed beneath the foot such that the first ray is not supported (Figure 10.15). If the heel is mobile it should adopt a valgus position. If it remains in a varus position it can be regarded as a fixed deformity.

Single-leg tip toe test

Take the patient to a wall so that they can lean on it for support. Normally, when a patient goes onto their tip toes the heel will go into varus and the medial longitudinal arch will be elevated. This is because of the 'windlass effect' whereby forced dorsiflexion of the MTP joint of the big toe tightens the plantar fascia and results in the medial arch raising and the heel going into varus.

When a patient is asked to tip toe on both and then one leg, normally they are able to do so. In the presence of a tibialis posterior tendon rupture, when asked to perform a double heel rise the affected foot remains in valgus rather than shifting into varus. The patient is unable to perform a single heel rise (Figure 10.16).

Testing the muscles around the ankle

Tibialis posterior: to test tibialis posterior function the foot is plantarflexed. From this position, resisted inversion is undertaken, which stresses the tibialis posterior (Figure 10.17). Palpate the tendon behind the medial malleolus.

Tibialis anterior: place the patient's ankle in maximum dorsiflexion and some inversion. Ask him or her to resist your attempt to plantarflex. Palpate the tendon at the front of the ankle (Figure 10.18).

Peroneus longus: to test for peroneus longus, place the patient's ankle in plantarflexion with the foot everted (the opposite of tibialis anterior). Ask the patient to maintain this position as the examiner pushes inwards (Figure 10.19). Feel the tendon behind the lateral malleolus.

Peroneus brevis: to distinguish between peroneus brevis and longus, the foot is placed in the neutral position and resisted eversion performed.

Silfverskiöld's test

This test is performed to determine whether gastrocnemius or soleus is the cause of reduced dorsiflexion of the ankle. Maximally dorsiflex the ankle first with the knee extended and then with the knee flexed to 90° (Figure 10.20). Because the gastrocnemius originates from above the knee, it tightens when

(a)

(b)

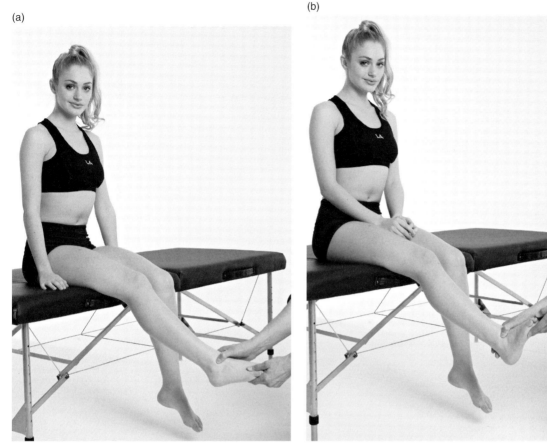

Figure 10.11 Anterolateral impingement test. **a** Apply thumb pressure over the anterolateral gutter with the foot in plantarflexion. This causes pain. **b** If the foot is then moved into dorsiflexion the pain intensifies, which is positive for synovial impingement.

the knee is extended and relaxes when the knee is flexed. If the loss of dorsiflexion is because of gastrocnemius tightness alone, then there will be reduced dorsiflexion with the knee extended. If there is no change of ankle dorsiflexion with knee flexion or extension, then the contracture is in both gastrocnemius and soleus.

Thompson's test

This is a test to determine whether there is a rupture of the Achilles' tendon. The patient lies prone on the couch with both ankles freely dangling over the end of the couch (Figure 10.21). Normally the resting tone of the gastrocnemius results in slight plantarflexion of the ankle. If there is a rupture of the Achilles' tendon the position of the ankle is more neutral. Squeeze the calf. In the presence of an intact tendon (sometimes also with a partial tear), there

will be passive plantarflexion at the ankle. If there is a complete tear, then there will be no response to the calf squeeze.

Anterior drawer test

This test is used to assess the anterior talofibular ligament of the lateral ligament complex. The patient is seated with the legs hanging over the side of the couch. The examiner grasps the heel with one hand and with the other hand holds on to the lower part of the leg. The examiner then pulls forward on the heel and pushes backwards on the lower leg (Figure 10.22). Laxity of the ligament is determined by increased anterior translation compared to the uninjured side. A soft endpoint can be appreciated. Sometimes in the anterolateral aspect of the joint, the dome of the talus tents under the skin.

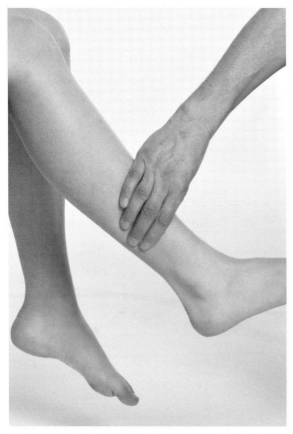

Figure 10.12 The 'squeeze test' for assessment of the distal tibiofibular syndesmosis.

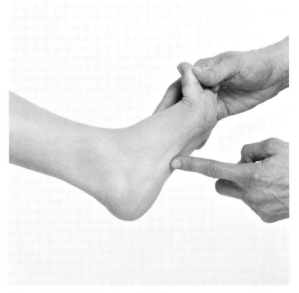

Figure 10.13 The 'windlass effect'. The great toe is maximally dorsiflexed, which tightens the plantar fascia and helps to reform the medial arch.

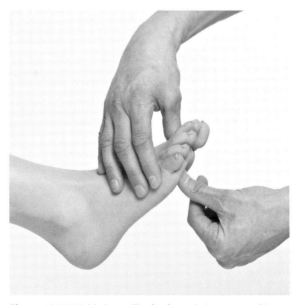

Figure 10.14 Mulder's test. The forefoot is being squeezed in a medial–lateral direction whilst at the same time pressure is applied from the plantar aspect of the foot under the affected web space.

Specific pathological conditions

Lesser toe deformities

Mallet toe – a flexion deformity of the distal interphalangeal (DIP) joint.

Hammer toe – a flexion deformity of the proximal interphalangeal (PIP) joint.

Claw toe – an extension deformity of the MTP joint and a flexion deformity of the PIP or DIP joint (Figure 10.23a).

In assessing a hammer toe deformity it is important to be able to differentiate between a fixed deformity at the PIP joint and a flexible deformity, because the treatment is influenced. To do this the PIP joint movements need to be examined with the long flexors of the toes relaxed. This can be accomplished by either plantarflexing the ankles or exerting upward pressure on the metatarsal heads (Figure 10.23b).

Cavovarus foot deformities

The commonest cause in the adult is Charcot–Marie–Tooth disease (hereditary motor and sensory neuropathy type I). It is autosomal dominant-inherited

(a)

(b)

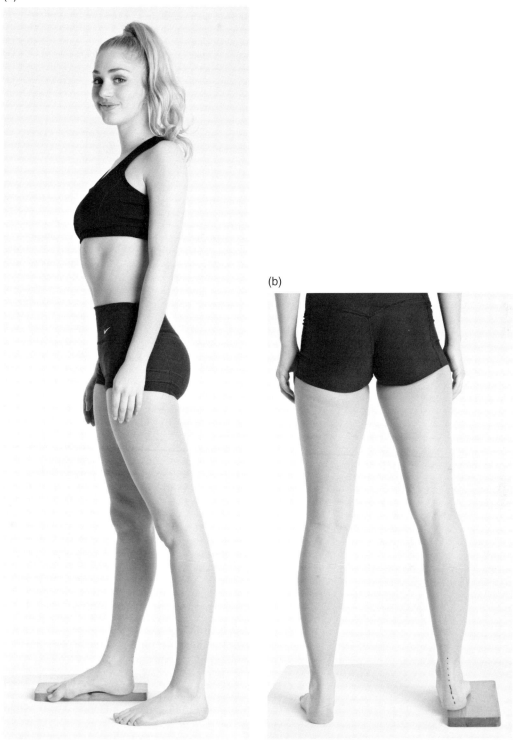

Figure 10.15 **a** and **b** The Coleman block test. The first ray and the great toe are placed off the edge of the block, allowing the heel to move back into a valgus position if there is no fixed deformity.

(a)

(b)

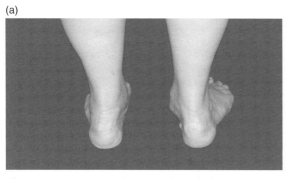 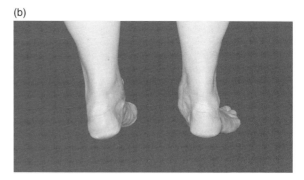

Figure 10.16 Tip toe test. This patient has a tibialis posterior rupture on the right side. **a** The heel is in valgus when standing. **b** When on tip toes note that the heel remains in valgus. This patient is unable to perform a single-leg tip toe test.

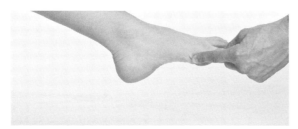

Figure 10.17 Testing for tibialis posterior.

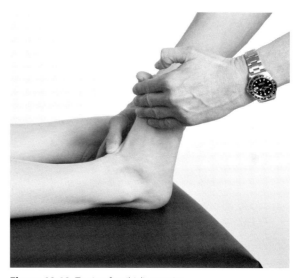

Figure 10.18 Testing for tibialis anterior.

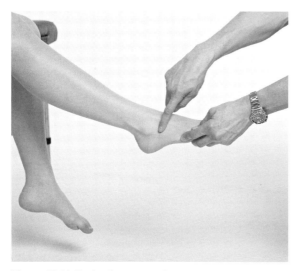

Figure 10.19 Testing for peroneus longus.

and typically presents in the second decade with symmetrical deformities. Asymmetrical cavovarus deformities are more typical of spinal dysraphism. Patients with Charcot–Marie–Tooth develop hindfoot varus, pes cavus, clawing of the toes and hands and

plantarflexion of the first ray (Figure 10.24). The Coleman block test will help to determine if the hindfoot varus is fixed or mobile.

Posterior tibial tendon disruption

This results from progressive degenerative change within the tendon. Symptoms range from pain and swelling along the medial aspect of the ankle to postural changes with loss of the medial longitudinal arch and hindfoot valgus. In patients with complete disruption of the tendon, more toes are visible when viewing the patient from behind (the so-called 'too many toes sign'[8]) resulting from increased abduction of the forefoot (Figure 10.25). This patient is unable to perform a tip toe test on the affected side. It is

(b)

(a)

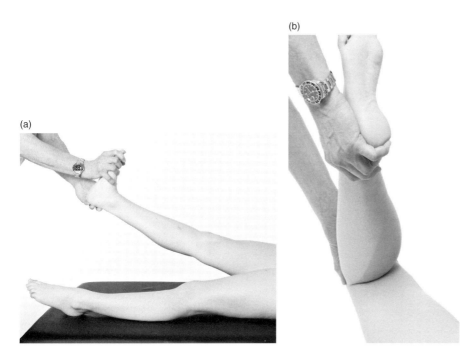

Figure 10.20 Silfverskiöld's test. This test is performed to determine if gastrocnemius is the cause of reduced dorsiflexion of the ankle. **a** Maximally dorsiflex the ankle first with the knee extended. **b** Repeat with the knee flexed to 90°.

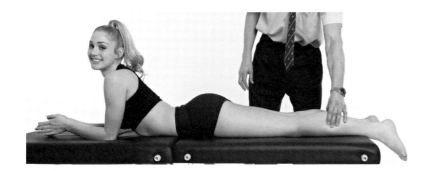

Figure 10.21 Thompson's calf squeeze test. Squeeze the calf with the patient in the prone position. Loss of passive plantar flexion of the ankle results from a complete rupture of the Achilles' tendon.

important to assess whether the hindfoot is fixed in valgus or corrects into varus and whether any compensatory forefoot position is fixed or mobile as this affects the treatment options.

Rheumatoid foot

This condition has a characteristic pattern of involvement. The hindfoot is often in valgus because of involvement of the subtalar joint and also the posterior tibial tendon. The midfoot is abducted, with loss of the medial longitudinal arch. There is clawing of the lesser toes and hallux valgus. On the plantar aspect

of the foot there are callosities over the prominent metatarsal heads (Figure 10.26).

Tarsal coalition

This condition usually presents in children when the fibrocartilaginous bar, which represents a failure of segmentation of the tarsal bones, ossifies. Patients complain of foot fatigue and hindfoot pain. In adults, recurrent ankle sprains may be a presenting feature. Tenderness is detected in the sinus tarsi with a calcaneonavicular bar, and medially around the sustentaculum tali with a talocalcaneal bar. The classical description of presentation with a tarsal coalition is one of a 'peroneal spastic flat foot'. The hindfoot is fixed in valgus with no inversion of the foot permitted. Not all patients with a coalition, however, have a fixed valgus deformity; some have neutral alignment and some have a varus deformity. The differential diagnosis of a fixed flat foot deformity in an adult includes septic arthritis, osteoid osteoma, inflammatory arthropathy, trauma and posterior tibial tendon disruption.

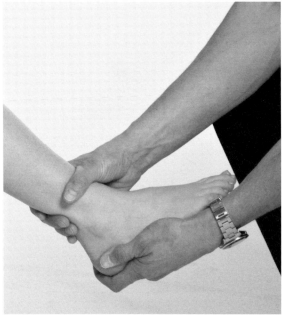

Figure 10.22 Anterior drawer test: to test for the anterior talofibular ligament.

Achilles' tendon disruption

The patient often describes being struck at the back of the leg. They are unable to perform a heel raise and a palpable gap is felt when placed supine. The patient may still be able to actively plantarflex their ankle because the long toe flexors are intact. However, squeezing the calf does not produce plantarflexion (Thompson's test).[9]

Peroneal tendon dislocation

This condition results from disruption of the superior peroneal retinaculum. It recurs in more than 50% of cases. In the chronic setting the patient describes a popping or snapping sensation lateral to the ankle. Movement of the foot and ankle from full plantarflexion and inversion to full dorsiflexion and eversion will often reproduce the dislocation. Pain and tenderness over the tendons is suggestive of a concomitant tear of the tendons.

(a)

(b)

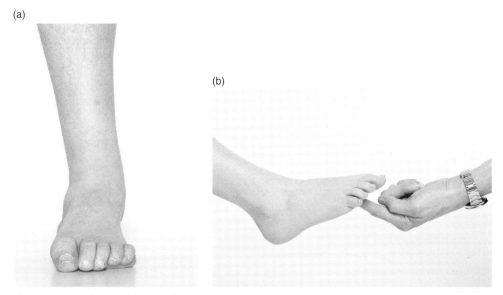

Figure 10.23 a Clawing of the toes of the forefoot. **b** To assess the flexibility of the PIP joints the long flexors to the toes need to be relaxed. This is achieved by elevating the metatarsal heads.

(b)

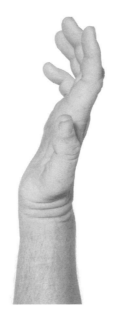

Figure 10.24 Charcot–Marie–Tooth disease. **a** Pes cavus and hindfoot varus. **b** Wasting of the intrinsic muscles and clawing of the hand.

(a)

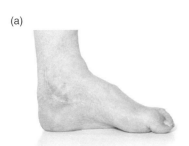

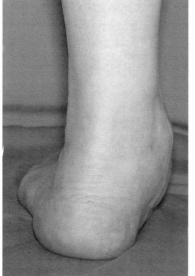

Figure 10.25 Tibialis posterior tendon rupture. Note the flattened medial arch, hindfoot valgus and 'too many toes'.

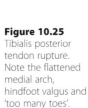

Figure 10.26 Rheumatoid foot. Note that the callosity is picked up only by deliberate inspection of the sole of the foot.

Ankle instability

Ankle instability can only be diagnosed with certainty using stress radiographs. Chronic instability is usually of the lateral ligaments (anterior talofibular ligament and the calcaneofibular ligament).

To test the calcaneofibular ligament an **inversion stress test (varus stress test)** is performed. With one hand, hold the ankle dorsiflexed to lock it. With the other hand, hold the calcaneus and invert it. Opening of the joint indicates laxity. Comparison with the other side may reveal a difference, but radiographs are needed to define whether the instability is occurring in the ankle, subtalar or both joints. The anterior drawer test (as described above) assesses the anterior talofibular ligament. In severe cases a suction sign develops just anterior to the lateral malleolus. Again, though, radiographs are required to confirm that the instability is occurring in the ankle.

Neurovascular assessment

This is undertaken after the three basic steps of inspection, palpation and movement have been completed. It is important to emphasize that many foot and ankle deformities result from neurological conditions. Inspection of the lumbar spine is therefore an integral part of examination of the foot and ankle. Similarly, in anyone complaining of neurological symptoms in the foot, it is also important to exclude lumbar nerve root tension. Assessment for clonus will distinguish between upper and lower motor neuron lesions. Assessment of sensation will help to identify patients at risk for ulceration and will also distinguish between conditions such as polio and spina bifida, both of which are lower motor neuron lesions. Motor testing should initially assess myotomal function and then concentrate on specific muscle groups, as directed by the history and examination. Assessment of the pulses concludes the initial general examination.

Although it is always important to consider the possibility of distant neurological disease affecting the foot and ankle, there are certain entrapment neuropathies around the foot and ankle that can be responsible for numbness, paraesthesiae and wasting.

Tarsal tunnel syndrome results from compression of the posterior tibial nerve in the tarsal canal. It is characterized by diffuse plantar pain associated with paraesthesiae and numbness. Percussion over the area of the entrapment may reproduce the symptoms, and palpation along the course of the nerve may reveal local causes such as lipoma, ganglion or exostosis. Physical findings must be supported with electrodiagnostic studies, especially if surgery is planned.

Deep peroneal nerve entrapment occurs most frequently beneath the inferior extensor retinaculum. It is often associated with trauma such as repeated ankle sprains. Patients complain of pain in the dorsum of the foot, with radiation into the first web space. Examination may reveal reduced sensation in the first web space and wasting of the extensor digitorum brevis.

Superficial peroneal nerve entrapment results from impingement of the nerve on the deep fascia as it exits the lateral compartment approximately 10 cm proximal to the ankle joint. Patients complain of pain in the lateral distal calf, which is often associated with numbness and paraesthesiae on the dorsum of the foot. Examination reveals point tenderness where the nerve exits the compartment. Where either deep or superficial peroneal nerve entrapment is suspected, the examiner must always palpate the common peroneal nerve around the neck of the fibula.

Other entrapment neuropathies have been described, such as sural nerve entrapment and entrapment of the first branch of the lateral plantar nerve. These must be considered once more common lesions have been excluded.

Foot and ankle terminology
N J Harris and M M Stephens

There still exists considerable ambiguity in the use of terms considering the joints of the human foot and their motions despite the efforts toward standardizing both of anatomists and clinicians.[10]

There are several reasons for this. The first is an embryological one. The foot is initially aligned with the leg, but rotates through 90° during development. This causes two of the axes of motion of the foot to do the same. Position and movement of the hindfoot are usually described with reference to the axes of motion of the leg, whilst the midfoot and forefoot (distal to Chopart's joint) are described relative to their embryological axes. If internal and external rotation of the midfoot and forefoot are replaced with pronation and supination, there become obvious similarities with upper limb movements.

Another reason for the confusion is that movements of the foot and ankle rarely occur in one plane. Combination patterns of movement have been described as early as 1889 by Farabeuf.[11] Inversion refers to plantarflexion, adduction and supination of the midfoot and forefoot, together with plantarflexion, adduction and internal rotation of the hindfoot. Eversion is the opposite, with dorsiflexion, pronation and abduction of the midfoot and forefoot together with dorsiflexion, abduction and external rotation of the hindfoot.

Summary

Summary of foot and ankle examination
Step 1 Stand the patient and look (include spine and hands as appropriate)
Step 2 Walk and look. Ask patient to tip toe (senior candidates consider doing single-leg tip toe test or Coleman's block test at this stage)
Step 3 Sit the patient Look at the sole of the foot, between the toes and look at shoes and walking aids
Step 4 Movements
Step 5 Palpation
Step 6 Special tests

The above sequence of **look, move, feel, special tests** flows best in examinations, especially for more senior candidates. **Look, feel, move, special tests** can be used as effectively by junior candidates. Palpation takes a long time to perform and may waste time in an examination as senior candidates may need to come to a provisional diagnosis following inspection and movements.

Stand

When standing the patient first look from the front, side and back and note any deformities or scars. Whilst looking from the back it is important to observe the position of the heel and to look for a 'too many toes sign' indicating tibialis posterior dysfunction. Always consider looking at the spine, as many foot and ankle problems are a manifestation of a neurological condition. Looking at the hands may give a clue to Charcot–Marie–Tooth in patients with pes cavus, while in patients with flat feet this may give an indication of underlying hyperlaxity (confirm by Beighton's scoring).

Walk

Walking will give clues to the diagnosis. Foot and ankle pathology will almost always affect gait.

Before sitting the patient down, more senior candidates may prefer to do relevant special tests here. For example, the tip toe test or, if the patient has a pes cavus, then the Coleman block test.

Sit patient

Sit the patient down and inspect the sole of the foot. Inspection of the foot is not complete without observing the sole of the foot and between the toes. This should be a cue for looking at the shoes and walking aids.

Move

Depending on the pathology, consider examining the joints from proximal to distal or distal to proximal. If the patient has possible ankle arthritis, then examine the ankle joint first. If the patient has a forefoot problem such as hallux valgus, then it may be more sensible to examine the distal joints first.

Feel

The foot and ankle joints are superficial and therefore tenderness in a particular area would mean pathology in that underlying structure. It would also lead the clinical examination on to the relevant special test; for example, tenderness in the third web space will lead on to Mulder's test, tenderness behind the medial malleolus would lead on to the tip toe test, etc.

Special tests

Coleman block test — A patient with a cavovarus foot would have a plantarflexed first ray. To assess the flexibility of the hindfoot, a block is placed beneath the foot such that the first ray is not supported. If the heel is mobile, then it should adopt a valgus position. If it remains in varus, then it is a fixed deformity.

Single-leg tip toe test — Ask the patient to hold onto something so that he or she does not overbalance. Ask the patient to stand on tip toes on both legs. Then ask him or her to repeat the manoeuvre on one leg. In the presence of a tibialis posterior tendon rupture the patient will be unable to do this on one leg.

References

1   Vanio K. The rheumatoid foot: a clinical study with pathologic and Roentgenological comments. *Ann Chir Gynaecol* 1956;**45**(suppl):1–107.

2   Coughlin MJ. Common causes of pain in the forefoot in adults. *J Bone Joint Surg (Br)* 2000;**82B**: 781–790.

3   Giannestras NJ. *Foot Disorders: Medical and Surgical Management*, 2nd edition. Philadelphia: Lea & Febiger, 1970.

4   Molloy S, Solan MC, Bendall SP. Synovial impingement in the ankle: a new physical sign. *J Bone Joint Surg (Br)* 2003;**85**:330–333.

5   Hopkinson WJ, St Pierre P, Ryan JB. Syndesmosis sprains at the ankle. *Foot Ankle* 1990;**10**:325–330.

6   Mulder JD. The causative mechanism in Morton's metatarsalgia. *J Bone Joint Surg (Br)* 1951;**33**:94–95.

7   Coleman SS, Chestnut WM. A simple test for hindfoot flexibility in the cavovarus foot. *Clin Orthop* 1977;**123**:60–62.

8   Churchill RS, Sferra JJ. Posterior tibial tendon insufficiency: its diagnosis, management and treatment. *Am J Orthopaed* 1998;**27**:339–347.

9   Thompson T, Doherty T. Spontaneous rupture of the tendon of Achilles: a new clinical diagnostic test. *J Trauma* 1962;**1**:126–129.

10 Sarrafian SK. *Anatomy of the Foot and Ankle*, 2nd edition. Philadelphia: Lippincott, 1993.

11 Farabeuf LH. *Précis de Manuel Operatoire: 816–847*. Paris: Masson, 1889.

Examination of the brachial plexus

Robert Winterton and Simon Kay

Full understanding of this topic is best achieved if the reader has knowledge of:

- Examination of the muscles around the shoulder girdle – see Chapter 2
- Examination of the peripheral nerves of the upper limb – see Chapter 6
- Anatomy of the brachial plexus – see below.

Anatomy

The brachial plexus is most commonly formed by the coalescence of nerve fibres from the C5, C6, C7, C8 and T1 spinal nerves (ventral primary rami). It emerges from the interscalene space, passing in the coronal plane laterally and caudally beneath the central third of the clavicle and above the first rib. It emerges from beneath the clavicle to pass deep to the muscles attached to the coracoid process before finally entering the axilla and upper arm from behind the lateral border of pectoralis major. It has important relationships throughout this course and these relationships bear upon the signs that may accompany injury to the plexus.[1]

Anatomical relationships

The skeletal relationships are most easily understood. The spinal column lies medial to the plexus and may lie in the same zone of trauma. The clavicle and first rib may each be fractured, and fracture of the first rib is associated with the dissipation of large amounts of kinetic energy. In exceptional circumstances, fracture of the scapula and clavicle may indicate that the arm has suffered a near avulsion injury: a brachiothoracic dissociation and that integrity of the skin envelope disguises substantial deep trauma.

Two important neural associations with the brachial plexus are the sympathetic nerves and the phrenic nerve. The sympathetic rami for the arm and face emerge from the T1 root immediately after it exits the cervical foramen. Avulsion of this root therefore carries a high incidence of Horner's syndrome: ptosis of the upper eyelid, meiosis of the pupil (smaller diameter), anhydrosis (loss of sweating on one half of the face: not easily demonstrated) and enophthalmos, which is not usually seen in the early stages (Table 11.1). The phrenic nerve arises from the C5 root as it lies on the medial scalene muscle and receives its main additional contribution from C4. Phrenic nerve palsy is therefore most likely to indicate avulsion of the C5 root with or without avulsion of the C4 root. In the latter case other signs of cervical plexus palsy may include numbness over the lateral neck and ear, or, rarely, trapezius palsy from involvement of the closely associated spinal accessory nerve.

The vascular relationships of the brachial plexus are most important, for not only do they provide evidence of collateral damage in cases of brachial plexus palsy, but that damage may itself be of great

Table 11.1 The features of Horner's syndrome

Meiosis
Constricted pupil in the absence of sympathetic tone
Anhydrosis
Unilateral loss of sweating in the face
Ptosis
Drooping of the upper eyelid resulting from loss of sympathetic tone in Müller's muscle
Enophthalmos
Relative atrophy of orbital contents

Examination Techniques in Orthopaedics, Second Edition, ed. Nick Harris and Fazal Ali. Published by Cambridge University Press. © Cambridge University Press 2014.

importance. The T1 spinal nerve arches cephalad and lateral to join C8 at the first rib and so form the lower trunk. The subclavian artery also crosses the first rib immediately anterior to the plexus and is intimately associated with the brachial plexus for the remainder of its course. The artery is therefore susceptible to injury in the same manner as the T1 nerve root, and penetrating or avulsion injuries of the plexus are often associated with vascular damage. Arterial injury is of greater significance than injury to the subclavian vein.

In summary, the roots of the brachial plexus lie between the scalenus anterior and medius muscles. The trunks lie in the posterior triangle of the neck. The divisions of the trunk lie behind the clavicle and at the outer border of the first rib. The cords lie medial, lateral and posterior to the axillary artery in the upper axilla.

Neural topography

The plexiform pattern of nerve coalescence and division is the result of the complex phylogenetic changes in the human limb as it evolved and assumed its current form. The pattern is variable and many find it difficult to recall. In fact it is in outline very simple. Three trunks bring nerve fibres to the plexus (the upper and lower are formed by the two most cephalad and the two most caudad roots) and each trunk divides into anterior and posterior divisions. These six divisions then regroup to form three cords, named for their relationship to the axillary vessels, and then each cord contributes to the four major nerves that enter the upper arm.

The radial nerve is formed mainly from the posterior cord, whilst the medial cord forms the ulnar nerve and part of the median nerve. The rest of the median nerve comes from that part of the lateral cord that does not become the musculocutaneous nerve.

Some key nerves leave the plexus at important points and these are indicated in Figure 11.1.

Knowledge of this neural topography helps the examining surgeon to establish an anatomical map of the parts of the plexus not functioning, and so to localize the lesion. In practice this localization is usually confined to estimating whether the injury is supraclavicular or infraclavicular, and how many roots are affected. The accuracy of identifying the structures injured in brachial plexus trauma from clinical examination is about 60%.

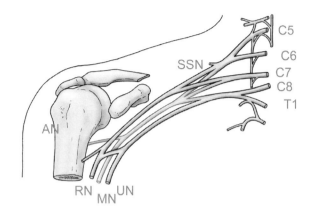

Figure 11.1 Brachial plexus with division into roots, trunks and cords together with branches. The roots C5 through T1 are shown. SSN, suprascapular nerve; UN, ulnar nerve; MN, median nerve; RN, radial nerve; AN, axillary nerve.

Examination

The examination should be considered in three phases, depending on how long has elapsed since the trauma:

- Immediately after trauma
- When the condition has stabilized
- The late stage.

Immediate aftermath of trauma

As with any trauma, the ATLS principles of screening for major life-threatening injury should be obeyed. In the case of a brachial plexus injury (BPI), the receiving surgeon should be especially alert to threats to the adjacent structures, i.e. the cervical spine, the great vessels and the thoracic cavity and contents. Having excluded life-threatening injury, the examiner should note the extent of the paralysis and sensory loss, and chart this accurately where possible. Often pain and distress will make this examination incomplete, but data should be recorded for future comparison. The examiner must be aware of the possibility of a Horner's syndrome in lower trunk injury, in which case the pupil inequality may be mistaken for a sign of cerebral injury. The vascular status of the limb should also be established and recorded, and evidence of subclavian artery rupture may include expanding supraclavicular haematoma.[2]

Routine investigation for all patients at this early stage should include cervical spine films and chest X-rays. In cases with extensive sensory loss in the arm, unappreciated fractures should be sought, especially

Table 11.2 Examination and investigations immediately post-trauma

Examination
- Exclude life-threatening injury (standard ATLS primary survey)
- Look for injury to adjacent structures
  - Cervical spine
  - Brain
  - Subclavian and mediastinal vessels
  - Thoracic cavity and contents
  - Appendicular skeleton
- Chart extent of sensory and motor loss as far as possible
  - Pinwheel, power, tendon reflexes
  - Horner's syndrome
  - Phrenic nerve
  - Examine the lower limb for long tract signs

Investigations
- Chext X-ray
  - Fractures
  - Widened mediastinum
  - Phrenic nerve paralysis
- Cervical spine X-ray
  - Fracture or instability
- Limb X-rays if insensate, especially wrist and forearm
- Angiography if vascular disturbance
- CT scan

of the wrist and forearm, where relatively subtle injuries can determine final outcome if undetected and untreated. Angiography may be indicated if vascular injury is suspected. The development of CT angiography has superseded contrast angiography in many units, and bony injury may be defined simultaneously where appropriate CT scanning protocols are employed (Table 11.2).

When condition stabilizes

When appropriate care has been given to the urgent treatment of bony, visceral or vascular injuries, the patient may be assessed in more detail. This is the first opportunity to detect and record important data that will have bearing in the days to come when deciding whether clinical signs are evolving. The use of a standard brachial plexus chart for recording the findings is useful but not essential. A simple scheme is to record sensory findings on a sketch of the limb (Figure 11.2) and to record motor findings by muscle group or by movement.

The aims of clinical examination of the brachial plexus

The aims of clinical examination of the brachial plexus are to:
- Determine the level of the lesion
- Determine the extent of the injury
- Determine the presence of any poor prognostic signs.

With regard to the level of the lesion, determine whether the injury is supraclavicular or infraclavicular.
- Supraclavicular lesions – roots and trunks affected
- Infraclavicular lesions – cords and branches affected.

For supraclavicular injuries it is important to determine whether the injury is preganglionic or postganglionic. Preganglionic means the lesion is proximal to the dorsal root ganglion.

Poor prognostic signs include:
- High-energy injury
- Older age
- Flaccid limb
- Painful anaesthetic limb
- Signs of preganglionic injuries. This includes Horner's syndrome, rhomboids or serratus anterior muscles affected.

Preganglionic lesions may be associated with long tract injuries to the spinal cord and have a poor prognosis for recovery. Preganglionic injuries are not reparable and require later nerve or muscle transfers. With postganglionic injuries there may be a chance of early repair.

To examine the **extent of brachial plexus lesion** competently, the candidate should have sound knowledge of the sensory and motor examination of the upper limb as described below.

General examination

Examine for signs of head injury, screen the cervical spine and look for a Horner's syndrome. Note coexisting injuries.

Where possible, the initial examination is facilitated if the patient is standing. The examiner should also stand and should begin by observation, inspecting the anterior and posterior aspects of the patient, noting posture, symmetry and signs of other injuries,

(a)

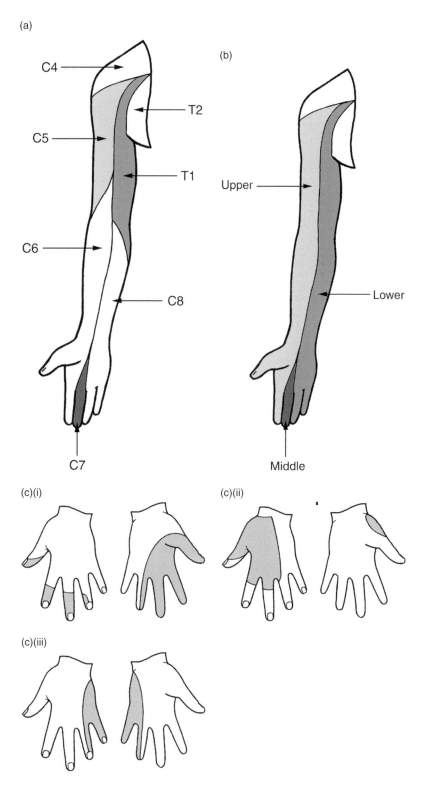

C4

C5

C6

C7

T2

T1

C8

(b)

Upper

Lower

Middle

(c)(i)

(c)(ii)

(c)(iii)

Figure 11.2 Sensory regions according to (**a**) roots; (**b**) trunks; (**c**) nerves: (i) median, (ii) radial, (iii) ulnar.

(a)

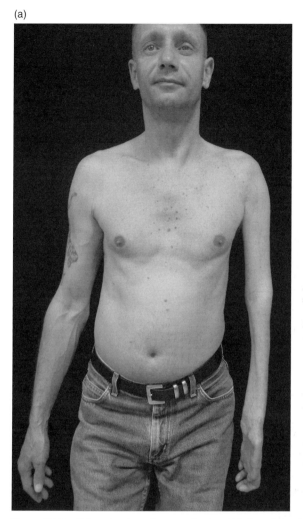

(b)

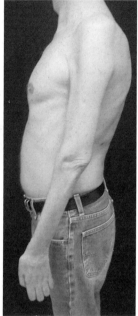

(c)

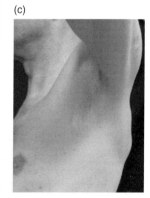

Figure 11.3 a This patient has a longstanding brachial plexus injury. Note the gross wasting, clawing of the hand, supination of the forearm and Horner's syndrome. **b** When looking from the side, wasting of the supraspinatus and infraspinatus is seen. **c** Remember to look into the axilla, especially for any scars from previous surgery.

as well as tropic changes and evidence of surgical treatment (Figure 11.3). If the patient is unable to stand, the reason should be determined, bearing in mind that avulsion of the roots of the plexus may be associated with long tract signs.

Horner's syndrome should be sought (Figure 11.4). Horner's syndrome indicates an injury to the sympathetic chain which is located near to the T1 root immediately after exiting from the foramen, and is usually associated with avulsion of this root.

Erb's palsy results from injuries to the upper part of the brachial plexus (C5, C6).[3] This can be the result of a difficult delivery at birth but can also occur after trauma to the head and shoulder where the two are

stretched apart. Pressure on the upper brachial plexus from a shoulder dislocation can result in an Erb's palsy. The classical features are loss of sensation in the arm as well as weakness of the deltoid, biceps and brachialis, resulting in an arm that hangs by the side internally rotated at the shoulder and with the forearm extended and pronated. This is called the 'waiter's tip' position (Figure 11.5).

Klumpke's palsy is a condition where the lower brachial plexus is injured (C8, T1).[4] It may be the result of a difficult vaginal delivery or trauma where there is forceful abduction of the shoulder such as hanging from a tree branch. The classic 'claw hand' shows the forearm supinated and the wrist and fingers

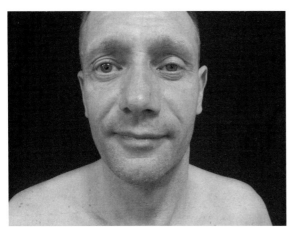

Figure 11.4 Horner's syndrome. This patient has ptosis, meiosis and enophthalmos. Anhydrosis completes the classic features of this syndrome.

flexed (Figure 11.6). Sensation may be lost in the ulnar forearm and hand.

Sensory examination

General palpation will reveal any areas of tenderness or fracture callus (Figure 11.7a). The sensory examination for different modalities is important but in the first instance the initial assessment is seeking areas of gross sensory loss, and the most expedient way to undertake this is with a pinwheel (pain or nociception: Figure 11.7b). This offers a measure of *threshold* assessment, and this may be supplemented by light touch using the examiner's own fingertips. In each case the perception of each stimulus should be compared to the uninjured side (if such exists), and the patient asked to comment on difference and similarity. Such examination may sometimes be usefully supplemented by examining other sensory modalities if a neuropraxia or conduction block is suspected, for in these injuries some fibres are preferentially affected, leading to a predictable loss of one modality before another (Figures 11.7c and 11.7d).

Because of the anatomical arrangement of the brachial plexus, traction (the commonest cause of damage) often produces a mixture of degrees of nerve injury. It is important to distinguish those nerves that have suffered a first-degree injury (neuropraxia), since recovery can be expected without intervention. In these cases certain characteristics are seen in the sensory loss. Firstly, it may change rapidly, and the densest loss may be only transient, placing great importance

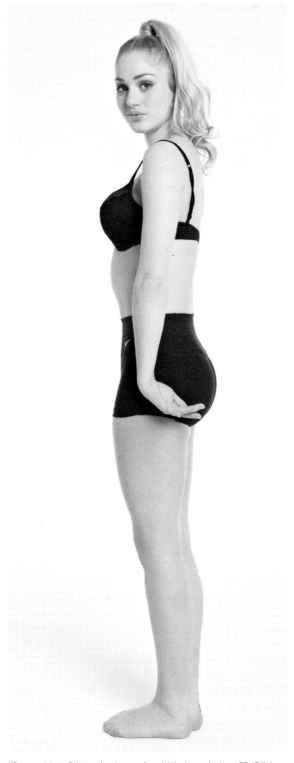

Figure 11.5 Erb's palsy (upper brachial plexus lesion; C5, C6) is demonstrated here with the shoulder internally rotated and the elbow extended and pronated, resulting in the 'waiter's tip' position.

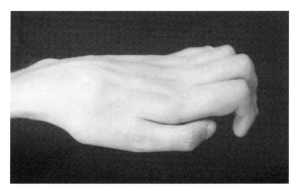

Figure 11.6 Klumpke's palsy (lower brachial plexus lesion; C8, T1) is manifested mainly in the hand with flexion of the fingers and wrist (claw hand). In addition, there is supination of the forearm.

on accurate recording of the signs from the first examination. Secondly, some modalities are more likely to be lost and are slower to recover, especially proprioception and light touch. Nociception, on the other hand, may be preserved, and this finding, in conjunction with the apparent preservation of sensibility in the presence of dense motor loss, should alert the examining surgeon to the likelihood of a first-degree nerve injury.

The sensory loss will then be plotted and will usually be found to correspond to the distribution of a root, a trunk or a nerve, allowing accurate assessment of the level of injury anatomically (Figure 11.8). The sensory recovery may be graded using the MRC system (Table 11.3) or, more usefully, with a descriptive system such as:

- No sensibility (i.e. anaesthetic)
- Pinprick sensibility recovered
- Moving touch felt
- Moving two-point discrimination of [] mm
- Static two-point discrimination of [] mm.

Autonomic function is often preserved in first-degree injury, but is lost acutely in all other degrees. Sweating should therefore be noted and recorded.

When assessing nerve injuries, a useful sign is Tinel's phenomenon. The principle underlying this sign is that the injured axon and the new growth cones of the regenerating nerve depolarize on mechanical stimulation. Percussion at the site of a significant nerve injury results in the patient perceiving tingling distal to the injury in the distribution of that nerve (whether motor or sensory). This is a reliable

localizing sign of nerve injury, but it should be remembered that this sign may also be present at the site of distal regeneration. Tinel's sign is not quantitative and the presence of a migrating Tinel's phenomenon indicates that some fibres are regenerating and its position tells how advanced that process is but does not indicate the eventual extent of recovery (Figure 11.9).

Because of the possibility of vascular damage, the pulse should also be palpated (Figure 11.10).

Motor examination

Examination of the motor system should then be undertaken. This is best conducted in a systematic manner from proximal to distal, and initially this focuses on muscle groups and their power. *A logical way of performing this examination is first to test the myotomes (roots), the nerves that come off the roots, the nerves that come off the trunks, the nerves that come off the cords and, finally, the terminal branches.*

In some groups, grading of power is useful, whilst other groups require more descriptive approaches. The commonest grading system for individual muscles is modified from that defined by Louisiana State University Medical Center (Table 11.4).

Each muscle group should be tested and each will provide information about level of injury in cases of avulsion.

The MRC grading system scores the whole limb and may not be as useful in describing the function after individual nerve injuries since it is most appropriately used for proximal limb muscle and is less descriptive or useful when applied to small muscles at the very periphery.

Root lesions

In practice, some patterns of injury are common and can easily be recognized. In isolated C5 root lesions the only loss is abduction of the arm (which may be weak rather than absent) and some sensory loss over the lateral aspect of the deltoid muscle (Figure 11.11a). This contrasts with an isolated axillary nerve palsy by the presence in the latter case of some activity in supraspinatus.

In C5, C6 root lesions a classic pattern with three components is seen and, once seen, is easily recognized. Here the shoulder abductors, the external rotators and the elbow flexors are paralysed

(a)

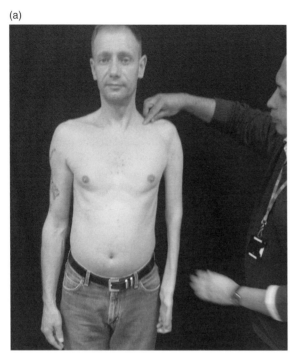

(b)

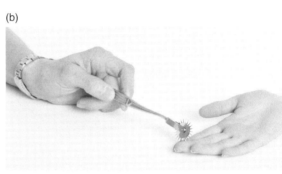

(d)

(c)

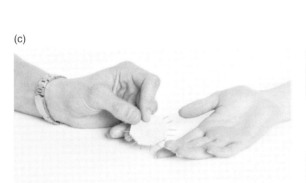

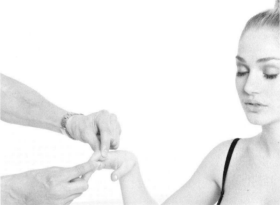

Figure 11.7 **a** Feeling starts with palpation for areas of tenderness or bony prominences such as fracture callus. **b** The use of a pinwheel to assess sensation. **c** Static two-point discrimination assesses the density of slowly adapting touch receptors, whereas moving two-point discrimination assesses rapidly adapting touch receptors. **d** Assessment of proprioception.

(Figure 11.11b). The arm is held internally rotated, and cannot be flexed at the elbow or abducted.

Combined C5, C6 and C7 root lesions are as above but with weak elbow extension and weak or absent wrist flexion and extension (Figures 11.11c, d).

Isolated or combined C7, C8, T1 root lesions have good proximal limb muscles but clawing in all digits

of the hand with weak flexion and extension of the fingers (Figures 11.11e, f).

The long thoracic nerve (serratus anterior) and the dorsal scapular nerve (rhomboids) come off the roots and should be assessed together with the myotomes because they may be injured together. Injury to these nerves indicates a preganglionic lesion.

Table 11.3 The MRC grading of sensation

S0	No sensation
S1	Pain sensation
S2	Pain and some touch sensation
S3	Pain and touch with no overreaction
S3+	Some two-point discrimination
S4	Complete recovery

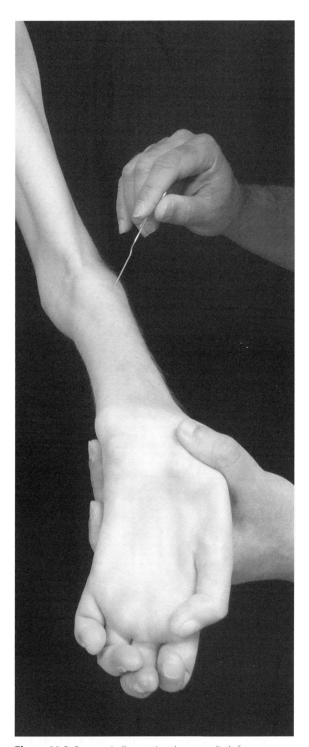

Figure 11.8 Systematically examine the upper limb for sensory deficit. Plot the areas of deficit on a simple line drawing to determine whether the lesion is at the level of roots, cords or terminal branches.

Starting with the patient facing away from the examiner, examine the rhomboids. These muscles approximate the two scapular borders and paralysis implies proximal damage to the C5 root since the nerve supply arises from this root almost immediately after it exits the cervical foramina (Figure 11.12a).

To test for serratus anterior the patient pushes against a wall with an outstretched arm, the fingers and palm pointing downwards on the wall. Scapular winging is observed if there is weakness from damage to the long thoracic nerve (Figure 11.12b).

Scapular stability is provided by a large number of muscles, prime amongst which are the rhomboids, serratus anterior and the trapezius. Paralysis of any of these three main muscles may result in an appearance of winging, which is therefore not always caused by long thoracic nerve palsy.

Trunk lesions

The muscles to be tested for trunk lesions are the trapezius and those supplied by the suprascapular nerve. The trapezius is supplied by the eleventh cranial nerve (spinal accessory), which is not part of the brachial plexus but lies in the posterior triangle of the neck and is therefore in close proximity to the trunks. The suprascapular nerve, which supplies the supraspinatus and infraspinatus, comes off the upper trunk.

The spinal accessory nerve is most commonly injured in the posterior triangle in the course of a node biopsy. The injury is often unappreciated despite the complaint of the patient. In part this is because the belief exists that trapezius is the primary shrugger of the shoulders. In fact that action is largely performed by levator scapulae, which can be felt contracting at the medial margin of the superior border of the scapula. Trapezius paralysis results in an inability to sustain abduction of the arm at 90° because the muscle acts as an elevator and stabilizer of the whole

Table 11.4 The Louisiana State University Medical Center grading of individual muscle power

Individual muscle grading	
0	No contraction
1	Flicker of contraction
2	Movement with gravity eliminated
3	Movement against gravity
4	Movement against gravity and some resistance
5	Full power

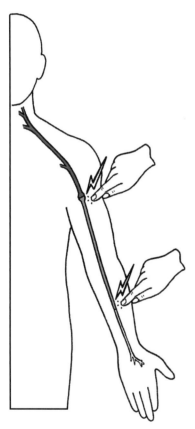

Figure 11.9 The principle of Tinel's phenomenon. Percussion over the site of nerve injury results in tingling or an electric shock sensation passing distally in the distribution of the nerve. A similar 'migrating Tinel's phenomenon' is found when percussing over the site of the advancing growth cones of regeneration.

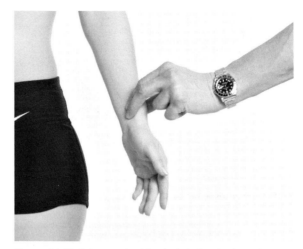

Figure 11.10 Palpation should include feeling for the pulse, as brachial plexus injuries may be associated with trauma to the subclavian or axillary vessels.

initiate abduction, whereas deltoid alone cannot. Conversely, supraspinatus can sustain abduction as can deltoid. In 90° of abduction, the most powerful extender of the glenohumeral joint is deltoid (posterior fibres). Weakness of supraspinatus may be distinguished from a rotator cuff tear with difficulty. External rotation is compromised and, if no contraction of supraspinatus can be felt, imaging of the joint or direct inspection may be required.

Cord lesions

Cord lesions may be associated with axillary artery damage as the cords are in intimate relationship with the artery. Feeling the brachial and/or radial pulse is essential.

The muscles to be tested for lesions involving the cords are the subscapularis (upper and lower subscapular nerves off the posterior cord), the latissimus dorsi (thoracodorsal nerve off the posterior cord) (Figure 11.14a) and the pectoralis major muscle (medial and lateral pectoral nerves off the medial and lateral cords) (Figure 11.14b).

Testing of these muscles is described in Chapter 2. Subscapularis is an internal rotator of the shoulder and is tested by **Gerber's lift off test** (Figure 11.14c). Shoulder adduction is achieved mainly with two large muscles (pectoralis major and latissimus dorsi) that derive their innervation from several roots each, and so offers little localizing information in terms of root involvement, but

shoulder girdle. However, if tested by shrugging the shoulder, the trapezius should be palpated to isolate it (Figure 11.13a).

The suprascapular nerve is assessed by testing supraspinatus (shoulder abduction) and infraspinatus (shoulder external rotation) (Figure 11.13b(i) and (ii)). These tests are described more fully in Chapter 2.

Distinguishing between weakness of supraspinatus and deltoid can be difficult. Supraspinatus can

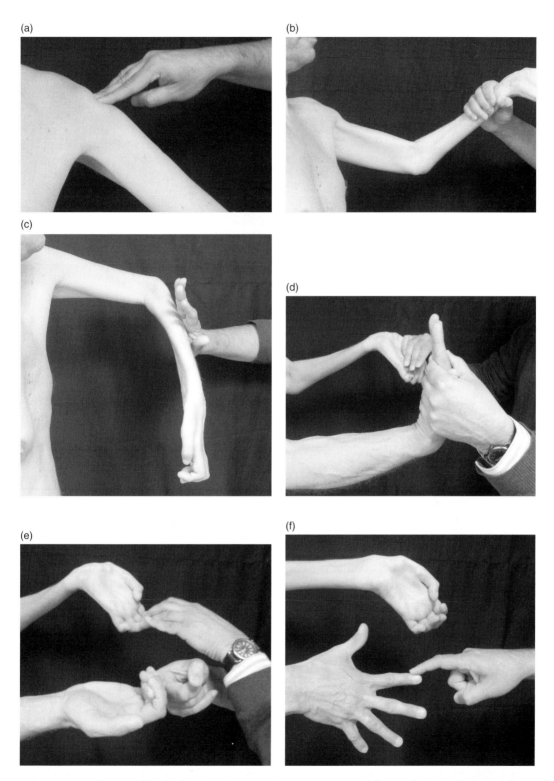

Figure 11.11 Assessing the roots of the brachial plexus by testing the myotomes. **a** C5; abduction of the shoulder. **b** C5, 6; flexion of the elbow. **c** C7, 8; extension of the elbow. **d** C6, 7; flexion and extension of the wrist. **e** C7, 8; flexion and extension of the interphalangeal joints of the fingers. **f** T1; intrinsic muscles of the hand. The first dorsal interosseous muscle of the right hand is being tested here.

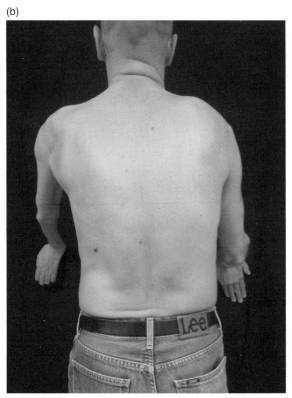

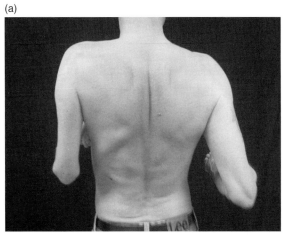

Figure 11.12 Assessing the muscles that are supplied by nerves coming off the roots of the brachial plexus. **a** Testing the rhomboids (dorsal scapular nerve, C5). Push the elbows backward and toward the midline against resistance and palpate the muscle. Also, the medial border of the scapula should move closer to the midline. Asymmetry between sides is suggestive of weakness. **b** Testing serratus anterior (long thoracic nerve, C5, 6 (7)). Patient pushes against a wall with outstretched arm, the fingers and palm pointing downwards on the wall. Look for scapular winging.

preservation of these muscles suggests involvement of the plexus distally, since the pectoral nerves emerge from the plexus early, and the thoracodorsal nerve emerges from the posterior cord. A qualitative appreciation of latissimus dorsi function can be obtained by grasping the anterior free borders of both muscles and asking the patient to cough, exploiting the role of this muscle as an accessory muscle of respiration.

Terminal branch lesions

The terminal branches of the cords are assessed in sequence. They are described in more detail in Chapter 6. It may be difficult to separate the loss of movements as a result of terminal branch injuries from that of root (myotome) injuries.

Shoulder abduction (C5): loss of abduction could be because of C5 root lesions or injuries to the axillary nerve (terminal branch of the posterior cord) where the deltoid is affected. To test for deltoid, passively abduct the shoulder to 90°, then extend it. Ask patient to resist as you push downwards on the arm (Figure 11.15a). Feel the muscle. This tests the posterior deltoid. The central and anterior fibres of the deltoid can be tested by placing the abducted arm in neutral and flexed positions, respectively. Deltoid function should be differentiated from supraspinatus (suprascapular nerve), especially in the position of forward flexion. The way to do this is to internally rotate the shoulder, thereby defunctioning the deltoid and isolating the supraspinatus.

The axillary nerve also supplies the teres minor muscle. This can be tested by looking for Hornblower's sign, as described in Chapter 2.

Elbow flexion (C5, C6): biceps brachii is innervated by the musculocutaneous nerve (lateral cord), as is the brachialis (predominantly musculocutaneous but some radial nerve laterally), whilst the brachioradialis is innervated by the radial nerve (posterior

(a)

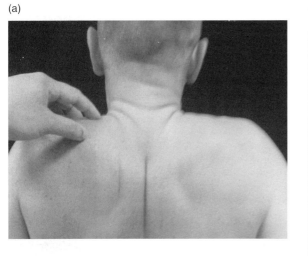

(b)(i)

(b)(ii)

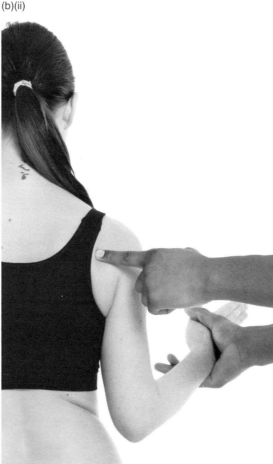

Figure 11.13 Assessing the muscles that are supplied by nerves off the trunks of the brachial plexus. **a** Testing trapezius. This muscle is supplied by the eleventh cranial nerve, but this nerve is located in the posterior triangle of the neck which can therefore be injured together with the trunks. To test, shrug the shoulders against resistance and palpate the muscle. **b** Test for supraspinatus and infraspinatus (suprascapular nerve off the upper trunk). Infraspinatus is shown here – elbow to the side and flexed 90°. (i) Ask patient to externally rotate and resist this movement. (ii) Feel the muscle.

cord). Elbow flexion should initially be tested without the effect of gravity. Further assessment should record range of elbow flexion and weight lifted or resistance (Figure 11.15b(i)).

Elbow extension (C7, C8) is predominantly triceps, from the radial nerve (posterior cord), and should be tested in a similar fashion to biceps (Figure 11.15b(ii)). Wrist extension is also predominantly C7 via the radial nerve (posterior cord).

Finger and thumb extension at the metacarpophalangeal (MCP) joints is predominantly C7, 8 (radial nerve) (Figure 11.15c). Flexion of the DIP joints of the thumb, index and middle fingers (via FPL and FDP) is from the median nerve (Figure 11.15d). The intrinsic muscles are T1 and essentially ulnar nerve (Figure 11.15e).

With the information from this examination the surgeon seeks to answer questions: where is the lesion

(a)

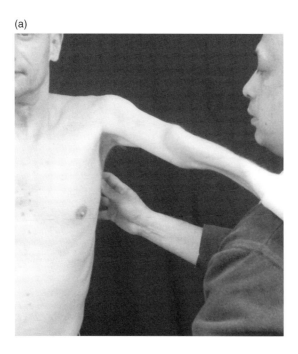

(b)

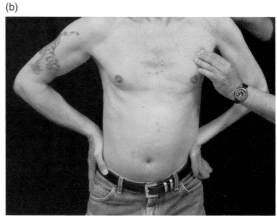

(c)

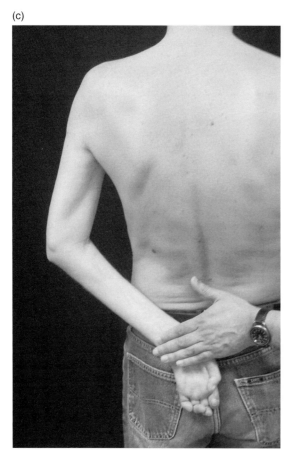

Figure 11.14 Assessing the muscles supplied by nerves arising from the cords of the brachial plexus. **a** Testing for latissimus dorsi (thoracodorsal nerve, posterior cord). Downward/backward pressure of the arm against resistance, as though climbing a ladder. Palpate muscle. This force may be exerted on the shoulder of the examiner, as shown here. **b** Testing for pectoralis major (medial and lateral pectoral nerves, medial and lateral cords, respectively). Hands on waist and squeeze inwards. Palpate the muscle. **c** Testing for subscapularis (upper and lower subscapular nerves, posterior cord). Gerber's lift off test. The arm is placed behind the back and the hand is passively positioned away from the body. Patients with subscapularis injuries are unable to maintain this position (lag sign). Power can be assessed by the examiner pushing against the patient.

(a)

(b)(i)

(b)(ii)

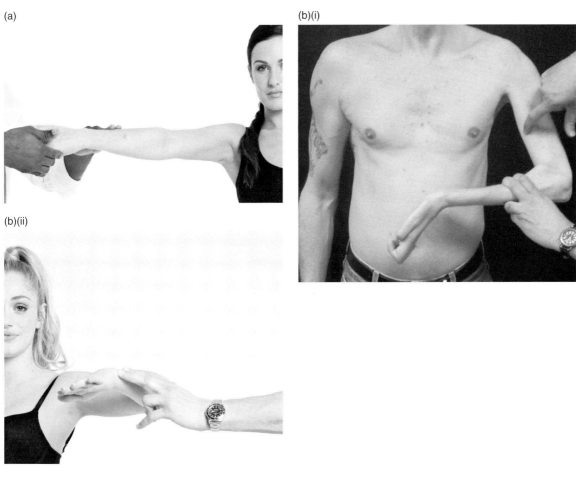

Figure 11.15 Assessing the terminal branches of the cords of the brachial plexus. **a Shoulder** – axillary nerve (terminal branch of the posterior cord); this is tested by abducting the shoulder against resistance to test the deltoid. **b Elbow** – (i) Musculocutaneous nerve (terminal branch of the lateral cord). Test the biceps brachii against gravity. Palpate the muscle. (ii) Radial nerve (posterior cord). Test the triceps (extension) with gravity eliminated. **c Hand** – radial nerve (terminal branch of posterior cord). Extension of MCP joint assessing extrinsic extensors. Quick screen: 'point your finger'. **d Hand** – median nerve (from terminal branches of medial and lateral cords). Flexion of the distal interphalangeal joint of index finger (flexor digitorum profundus) and interphalangeal joint of thumb (flexor pollicis longus). Quick screen: 'OK sign'. **e Hand** – ulnar nerve (terminal branch of medial cord). Interosseous muscles of the hand. Quick screen: 'cross your fingers'.

and how extensive is it? Some investigations may help in answering these questions.

Investigations

Imaging

Radiographs may already have given some information about adjacent skeletal injuries that provide clues to the extent of injury. Myelography may be employed to show myeloceles (presumptive evidence of intradural injury, which may or may not be complete) or define the intradural rootlets or their

absence. Combined with a CT scan the sensitivity of this investigation is increased, but false positives and negatives can occur in up to 5% of cases. MRI studies alone have yielded similar results in some units.

Electrical studies

Electrophysiology adds little to the clinical findings in the cooperative awake patient at this stage unless it is necessary to exclude the possibility of a conduction block or neuropraxia. In the unconscious polytrauma patient such studies may be useful.

(c)

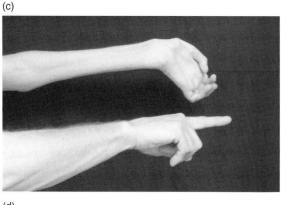

(d)

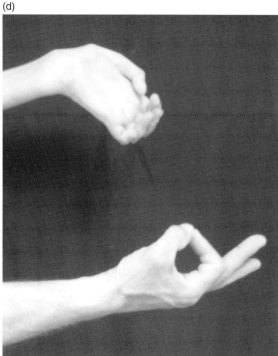

(e)

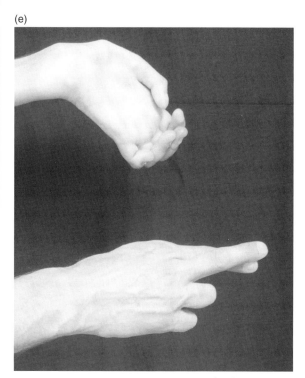

Figure 11.15 (cont.)

Treatment

The key question at the early stage (assuming that other injuries permit) is whether or not surgery is immediately indicated. Opinions vary on the precise indications for surgery, but some observations may be made.

Firstly, the primary intent of surgery is diagnosis. No clinical inference or imaging study will substitute for a direct examination of the plexus from foramina to axilla by an experienced surgeon. This is, however, a considerable undertaking and should be done only in the expectation of finding pathology that can then be immediately treated. Thus the examination aims to predict such pathology and to shape a plan for treatment that can be discussed prior to surgery and completed at surgery.

The late stage

Faced with a patient many months after injury the surgeon will have to answer different questions. The results of exploration and repair are poorer after 6 months and, in general, not worthwhile for restoration of motor function in adults after 1 year, although some improvement in sensibility may occur. At this stage the surgeon will be examining the patient with a view to secondary reconstruction, and the options here are numerous.

In general they consist of osteotomy, arthrodesis, tendon transfers and, in some cases, nerve transfers to power free-functioning muscle transfers. For these reasons the surgeon will need to evaluate the degree of recovery and determine whether further recovery is taking place. He or she will be interested in the function of the hand and its supporting structures and in determining whether the injury is primarily upper root or lower root. In upper root palsy the hand may function very well but the patient may lack the vital positioning qualities of a stable shoulder, together with external rotation and elbow flexion. In the converse situation, absent lower root function may leave good shoulder or elbow function with little hand use, raising doubts about the value of complex proximal reconstruction.

Summary
Fazal Ali and Joe Garcia

> ## Summary of the brachial plexus examination
>
> ### Step 1
> Stand the patient and look
> - Inspect the position in which the arm is held. Look for scars, wasting and for the presence of Horner's syndrome
>
> ### Step 2
> Feel
> - Over bony areas
> - Sensation – dermatomes and peripheral nerves
> - Feel the pulse and for sweating
>
> ### Step 3
> Move
> - Assess the myotomes of the upper limb
> - Assess the muscles supplied by the nerves off the roots of the brachial plexus
> - Examine the muscles supplied by the nerves off the trunks of the brachial plexus
> - Examine the muscles supplied by the nerves off the cords of the brachial plexus
> - Examine the muscles supplied by the terminal branches of the brachial plexus

The aims of clinical examination of the brachial plexus are:

1. Determine the level of the lesion (supraclavicular or infraclavicular).
2. Determine the extent of the injury (sensory and motor deficit).
3. Determine the presence of any poor prognostic signs (preganglionic injuries).

To examine competently for the level and extent of a brachial plexus lesion, the candidate should have sound knowledge of the following aspects of the clinical examination.

Sensory
- Dermatomes of the upper limb
- Cutaneous nerve supply to the upper limb such as area supplied by radial nerve, median nerve, ulnar nerve and musculocutaneous nerve, etc.

Motor
- Myotomes to the upper limb
- Demonstrate power in the muscles of the shoulder girdle
- Demonstrate muscles of the rotator cuff
- To be able to examine radial nerve, ulnar nerve and median nerve.

Once the candidate is proficient in doing the above, then examination of the brachial plexus injury is much easier. The system for the examination is **look, feel, move**.

Look
- On standing, look at the position in which the patient holds the arm. It may be adducted and internally rotated, as in upper trunk lesions (Erb's paralysis) with the 'waiter's tip' position
- There may be a clawed hand, as in lower trunk lesions (Klumpke's paralysis)
- Look for scars, including in the axilla. These may be surgical scars or scars related to a penetrating injury
- Look for wasting of the muscles of the shoulder girdle in the upper limb
- Look for Horner's syndrome, which includes ptosis, myosis, anhidrosis and enophthalmus. Horner's syndrome is damage to the sympathetic chain, which is in close proximity to the nerve roots and signifies the possibility of a preganglionic lesion

- If the patient cannot stand, then the long tracts of the spinal cord may be damaged as these are close to the roots of the brachial plexus.

Feel

- Feel over bony prominences for previous fractures, especially clavicle and scapular fractures
- Test the dermatomes and the area supplied by the peripheral nerves. A dermatomal pattern of loss of sensation may indicate root or trunk injuries, whereas a peripheral nerve pattern of sensory loss may indicate lesions of the cord or the terminal branches of the brachial plexus
- It is important also to feel the pulse in the upper limb, as the brachial plexus is closely related to the subclavian and axillary arteries
- Feeling for sweating on the side is an important sign, as this sign may be preserved in the presence of a neuropraxia.

Move

- **Myotomes**, i.e. C5/6/7/8 and T1 of the upper limb
- The muscles supplied by nerves arising off the **roots:**

Dorsal scapular nerve (C5) – rhomboids
Long thoracic nerve (C5, 6, 7) – serratus anterior

- Muscles supplied by nerves arising from the **trunks:**

Suprascapular nerve (C5/6) upper trunk – supraspinatus and infraspinatus
Trapezius can be tested to indicate trunk lesions because the eleventh cranial nerve lies in the posterior triangle of the neck near to the trunks

- Muscles supplied by nerves arising from the **cords:**

Medial and lateral pectoral nerve (medial and lateral cord) – pectoralis major
Thoracodorsal nerve (posterior cord) – latissimus dorsi
Upper and lower subscapular nerve (posterior cord) – subscapularis

- Muscles supplied by the **terminal branches** of the brachial plexus:

Radial nerve, median nerve, ulnar nerve, axillary nerve and musculocutaneous nerve.

The accuracy of assessing a brachial plexus injury by clinical examination is about 60%.

References

1 Moore KL, Agur AM. *Essential Clinical Anatomy*, 3rd edition. Baltimore: Lippincott Williams & Wilkins, 2007.

2 Midha, R. Epidemiology of brachial plexus injuries in a multitrauma population. *Neurosurgery* 1997;**40**:1182–1189.

3 Peleg D, Hasnin J, Shalev E. Fractured clavicle and Erb's palsy unrelated to birth trauma. *Am J Obstet Gynecol* 1997;**177**:1038–1040.

4 Shoja MM, Tubbs RS. Augusta Déjerine-Klumpke: the first female neuroanatomist. *Clin Anat* 2007;**20**:585–587.

Further reading

Garcia J, Ali F. Clinical examination of the brachial plexus. *Chesterfield and Sheffield FRCS(Tr&Orth) Clinical Course Manual*, 2012, pp. 42–45.

Orthopaedic examination techniques in children

James A. Fernandes

Paediatric orthopaedic examination is an art, and the success of the consultation relies on the surgeon's ability to communicate with the parents and the child. Most children who are referred do not require surgery, and time is spent on reassuring the anxious parents or guardian of the normal variations in the development of the child. Quite often, observing the child during the consultation with the parents and a thorough general examination give the clues in making a clinical diagnosis.

The paediatric consulting area should be child-friendly, with toys and ample space for the child to play and for the surgeon to observe. Gaining the confidence of the child is crucial, as well as being warm and patient with the parents who are anxious and concerned. The initial interview should include introductions, as it is important to know the accompanying adults apart from the parents. They could be carers, guardians, grandparents or physiotherapists, and valuable information could be gained. History should be gained from the parents as well as the child, for, not infrequently, it could be conflicting. Clinical history skilfully obtained is the key to diagnosis, and a methodical examination of the child depending on the symptoms and age confirms your initial impression.

History
General

The history usually starts with some statistical and demographic data, followed by the presenting complaint. Common complaints are of deformity, limp, gait abnormalities, weakness (generalized or localized), pain, swelling or stiffness of joints. It is worthwhile asking the older child about his or her symptoms. The chronological order of the mode of

onset, time period, severity, disability, and aggravating and relieving factors should be noted. History of trauma should be investigated thoroughly for its aetiological significance. Since many of the symptoms arise from the musculoskeletal system that is concerned with support and locomotion, questions should be directed to establishing a relationship of symptoms to physical activity.

Prenatal history is of paramount importance. History of unusual incidents, vaginal bleeding, infections such as rubella in the first trimester give clues in the congenital afflictions. Maternal history of diabetes mellitus, toxaemia and syphilis are associated with abnormalities at birth. Fetal movements in later pregnancy can be reduced in arthrogryposis multiplex congenita and Werdnig–Hoffman disease. In the birth history, the type of presentation, birth weight and Apgar score should be sought. Further perinatal-related questions, including jaundice, should be described.

Developmental history for physical and mental milestones should be sought (Table 12.1). Upper limb developmental functions and handedness is important. Information about school performance and physical activities give further insight. This is usually followed by a systemic review, including unusual bruising, easy bleeding and allergies. Past illnesses, hospitalizations and family history completes the orthopaedic history.

Specific
Limp and gait disturbances

Did the child start limping with complaints of pain? How was the onset? Acute transient synovitis of the hip is usually associated with a history of upper respiratory tract infection 7–14 days before the episode. The pain could be in the knee, thigh or hip

Examination Techniques in Orthopaedics, Second Edition, ed. Nick Harris and Fazal Ali. Published by Cambridge University Press. © Cambridge University Press 2014.

Table 12.1 The important developmental milestones

Age	Motor	Language
3 months	Lifts head up when prone	Vocalizes without crying
6 months	Head steady when sitting	Smiles and laughs
9 months	Pulls self to stand	Non-specific words (da-da, ma-ma)
1 year	Walks with one hand support	Two or more words
14 months	Walks without support	
2 years	Runs forward	Three-word sentences
3 years	Jumps in place	Knows whether boy or girl
4 years	Balances on one foot	Counts three objects correctly
5 years	Hops on one foot	Names four colours
6 years	Skips	

because of the peculiarity of the same nerve supply. Was there any history of trauma? Post-traumatic avulsions of apophyses around the hip produce a painful limp. Where is the pain? Adolescent children developing slipped capital femoral epiphyses more commonly present with aching pain, more often in the knee than the groin, hip or thigh. This may be associated with an abnormal out-toeing gait, especially with chronic slip. In the acute slip, there may be sudden severe pain with difficulty in weightbearing. Children in the age group of 4–8 years are more likely to have the initial presentation of Perthes' disease. Painful limp and difficulty weightbearing with constitutional and systemic symptoms should be urgently assessed for septic infection of joints, commonly the hip or in bone.

Was the limp noticed from walking age? Painless limp with short leg can be seen in late presentation of a dislocated hip, and painful limp at the end of the day could be a symptom of adolescent acetabular dysplasia or developmental coxa vara. Abnormal asymmetrical gait could be a feature of a neurological presentation. Abnormal posturing and gait abnormalities might be the only symptoms in rare spinal cord tumours and even in lumbar discitis.

Deformities

Flexible flat feet are usually familial, with some family history of ligamentous laxity. Is there a progressive deformity of toes and feet? Pes cavus warrants a family history to rule out hereditary sensorimotor neuropathy, Friedreich's ataxia or other disorders. Painful flat feet in adolescence could be the first presentation of tarsal coalitions or inflammatory arthropathies. The former can also present with frequent ankle sprains.

Intoeing gait is one of the common complaints (Figure 12.1). If present from walking age and bilateral, usually the common causes are metatarsus

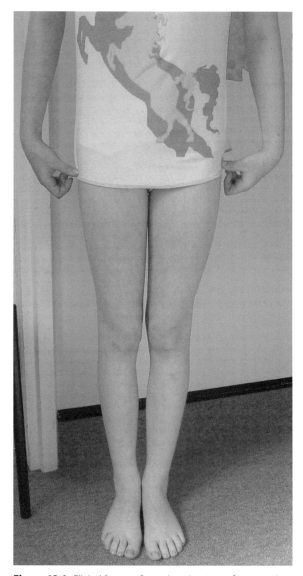

Figure 12.1 Clinical features for an intoeing type of presentation. Note that the patellae point inwards.

adductus, persistent excessive femoral anteversion or internal tibial torsion, with the latter two remodelling 95% of the time by age 7–9 years. Any unilateral intoeing or outtoeing needs to be further assessed and, if rapidly progressive, pathological conditions such as neurological, tumour, infection and congenital causes should be considered.

Bow legs and knock-knees are common deformities for which parents ask for consultation. Ask about the progression of these deformities? Quite often they are physiological and, if severe, need to be investigated further. Nutritional rickets is one of the commonest causes in the developing and third world, whereas questions relating to renal and familial rickets should be asked when such deformities are seen in the developed world. Any asymmetric deformity could have an underlying cause. Consider Blount's disease in an Afro-Caribbean child with proximal tibial varus.

Limb length discrepancy

Limb length discrepancy, with or without associated deformities, could have various causes. When was it first noticed? Was it noticed at birth and is it progressing? Is one shoe size smaller than the other? Was it noticed with a unilateral tip toeing gait at walking age, suggesting a possibility of a late presentation of developmental dysplasia of the hip (DDH)? Is the child using a shoe raise? Does the child complain of any backache? Is one limb larger in length and girth as in hemihypertrophy? Is there a family history of neurofibromatosis? Was there any history of trauma or injury to the growth plates? Was there any history of infection of a joint or bone? These could cause discrepancy with deformity. A positive family history for deformity may indicate a syndrome or some skeletal dysplasias.

Weakness

Localized weakness in the lower or upper limbs is rare and could be due to neuropraxias after injury or to any bony lumps pressing on nerve structures, as in hereditary multiple exostoses. Adolescents may occasionally present with back pain, sciatica and weakness of toe dorsiflexors in acute disc protrusion. Generalized weakness could be a feature of metabolic bone disorders. Boys who complain of being easily tired and who are toe walkers should be investigated for muscular dystrophy with a simple test for creatine phosphokinase. Neuromuscular conditions like myopathies and others may present with floppy baby, slow developmental milestones, awkward gait and weakness. Space-occupying lesions in the base of the skull or spinal cord may have unusual presentations of weakness with abnormal gait.

Obstetric birth palsies can present with deformities, abnormal posture and partial or total loss of movements of the upper limb. Was there a large head or breech presentation? Was there a history of difficult labour? When was it first noticed and is there any progress in recovery of movements?

Swelling

When did the swelling appear and is it getting larger? Is there pain and has it progressed in size rapidly? These could be localized swellings or generalized around joints. Soft tissue swellings are usually slow growing and benign like ganglias, and are usually pain-free. Any swelling associated with pain should be evaluated for soft tissue sarcomas. Does the swelling fluctuate in size? Haemangiomas, which are common around the knee, give a history of fluctuation in size as well as the semimembranous bursa at the back of the knee. Bony lumps are usually in the metaphyseal regions of the long bones and could be multiple, as in hereditary multiple exostoses. The practitioner should ask about any associated pain, functional loss or compromise in joint movement.

Swelling of joints with associated joint stiffness needs further questioning regarding the onset, periodicity, small or big joints and whether there was a rash or erythematous reaction. Family history of inflammatory conditions should be part of the history-taking. Single joint affections need to be further explored for any foci of infection and systemic symptoms like pyrexia.

Scoliosis

History should include whether this was noticed at birth or was associated with any other congenital condition or syndrome. If later, when was it noticed? Is it progressing rapidly and is it associated with other chest cage deformities? Is there any associated pain? Painful scoliosis is a presenting syndrome for an underlying spinal cord or cauda equina tumour as well as bony tumours of the spine such as osteoid osteoma or osteoblastoma. Night pain could be an ominous symptom for either an infection or a tumour. Ask for family history of neurofibromatosis? Patients with other neuromuscular conditions like cerebral palsy and Duchenne muscular dystrophy also develop scoliosis.

Examination

Examination of the child starts from the child entering the room and observation takes place while the history is taken. Many clinical signs can be picked up from the parents giving clues in the genetically inherited conditions like neurofibromatosis, flat feet and scoliosis. The child should be undressed appropriately and in stages if required. Babies below the age of 6 months can be examined on the couch whereas the toddler and infant can remain on the parent's knee until confidence is gained. Respecting the older child's modesty is vital. Examining the orthoses or shoewear may give further information.

General

Inspection of the facies may give valuable clues in syndromic conditions and other skeletal dysplasias. When noted, dysmorphic features need to be of significance; looking at the parents' facies may also help. Blue sclerae can clinch the diagnosis of osteogenesis imperfecta and mongoloid features for Down's syndrome. Asymmetric sizes of pupils, i.e. miosis, with or without ptosis, is a sign of Horner's syndrome (Figure 12.2). The height of the child should be recorded, as well as the heights of the parents, both standing and sitting. Metabolic disorders or skeletal dysplasias should be considered where there is short stature associated with lower limb deformities. Anthropometric measurements should include head and chest circumference, span, segmental lengths and ratios of the different segments. Any asymmetry in the body proportions of each side, including the tongue, should be sought, especially hemihypertrophy. Hemiatrophy with history of low birth weight may instigate an investigation for Russell–Silver syndrome.

Standing examination in general

Examine from the front, side and the back; assess the standing posture and the normal curves of the spine. Look at the level of the shoulders and contour, level of the anterior superior iliac spines (ASIS) and symmetry. A plumbline held at the centre of the occiput should pass through the natal cleft. Frontal and sagittal balance should be assessed. Look for external spinal markers of dysraphism such as a dimple, a tuft of hair, naevus or a lipoma. In neurofibromatosis, look for café-au-lait spots, axillary or inguinal freckling and neurofibromas. Are there any vascular markings, as in Klippel–Trenaunay syndrome, or other blemishes? Note whether there are any defects of the limbs. If the creases of the limbs are not matching and the pelvis not square, use blocks to lift the shorter side and level the iliac crests.

The general alignment of the lower limbs is then assessed for genu varum or genu valgum (Figure 12.3), and this can be quantified with graduated wooden

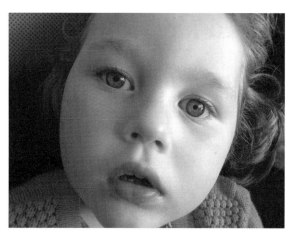

Figure 12.2 Small pupil on the left as seen in Horner's syndrome.

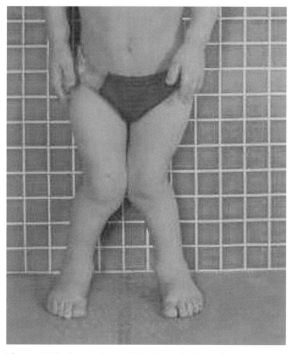

Figure 12.3 Genu valgum deformity at the knees in pseudoachondroplasia.

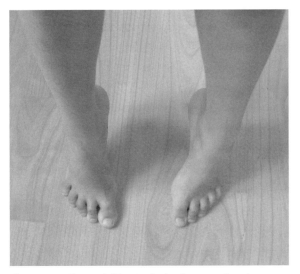

Figure 12.4 The medial longitudinal arch on standing tip toes.

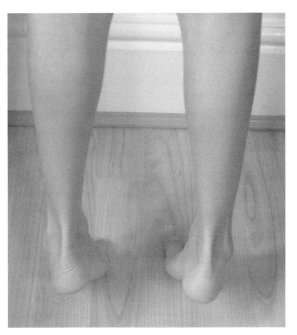

Figure 12.5 The heels going into varus on standing tip toes.

triangles at the intercondylar or intermalleolar levels. The reference is the knee, and the child should be made to stand with the patellae facing straight forward, medial malleoli touching each other when varus and the medial femoral condyles touching each other when valgus. The feet should be assessed for any cavus, flat footedness and hindfoot alignment. Standing on tip toes should lead to the formation of a robust medial longitudinal arch (Figure 12.4) and the heels should go into neutral or varus (Figure 12.5). The hindfoot should normally be in 6–7° valgus to the long axis of the calf when standing.

Gait

Next, ask the child to walk in a straight line and look for any abnormal upper limb movements suggesting hemiplegia, athetoid or spastic movements. Look at the foot progression and knee progression angles, which give the degree of intoeing or outtoeing, and the level at which they arise. Look at the way the foot strikes the ground and whether a normal heel-to-toe type of gait is present. Assess knee extension on heel strike and flexion in swing. Look at the pelvis in all three planes.

Limp

Limp can be described as any asymmetrical movement of the lower limbs. A limp can be due to pain (when it is called antalgic) or result from limb length discrepancy, instability at the hip or neurological causes.

An **antalgic gait** is when the stance phase of the affected limb is hurried with a quick swing phase of the opposite limb. It can result from any painful cause, from the sole of the foot to the pelvis. One can therefore broadly classify any gait as antalgic or non-antalgic gait and then specify.

Short-limbed gait is when the shoulder dips down on the shorter side on stance phase, as seen in children with longitudinal deficiencies.

The **Trendelenburg gait** is due to failure of the abductor mechanism on the affected side to hold the pelvis level in the stance phase, with a compensatory sway of the ipsilateral shoulder, classically called the 'lurch', thereby shifting the centre of gravity to the midline. This produces a characteristic waddling or swaying, which becomes very dramatic in bilateral conditions, e.g. bilateral neglected congenital dislocation of the hip (CDH), bilateral coxa vara.

High stepping gait is seen with a foot drop when the dorsiflexors are ineffective at the ankle in achieving foot clearance; this produces the slapping foot, as seen in neurological disorders such as hereditary sensorimotor neuropathy. This abnormality is seen in the swing phase.

Toe walking or **tip toe gait** is when the child's initial contact is with the forefoot and the contralateral foot follows the same. This is seen in habitual tip toe walkers with or without a tight heel cord and could be the earliest presentation of Duchenne muscular dystrophy. Any increase in tone of the limbs should suggest features of cerebral diplegia.

When the triceps surae is weak, a **calcaneus gait** is seen with lack of push-off and, when severe, is called the **'peg' gait**, as the stance phase remains on the heel throughout. This is often seen in lower motor neuron paralytic conditions and in overcorrected clubfeet after radical surgery.

The stiff knee produces a limp, and the pelvis is either hiked to clear the limb or the patient can circumduct the leg.

When the quadriceps is weak, patients compensate by 'back kneeing' to prevent the knee from collapsing, and fixed equinus helps to achieve this. Some children with paralytic conditions will use the hand to push the front of the thigh backwards to achieve back kneeing, otherwise called the **'quadriceps'** or **'hand-to-knee' gait**.

Neurological gaits are of various types and can be combinations. Spastic gait is of equinus at the ankle, flexion at the knee and hips, with adduction and internal rotation of the lower limbs, producing dragging or scraping characteristics and, when static, has the 'jump' posture. Scissoring of the lower limbs can be seen when there are adduction and internal rotation deformities at the hips. The **crouch gait** is when the triceps is weak and the gait lacks push-off with the ankles in dorsiflexion in stance.

Ataxic gait is associated with a broad base and, when severe, the feet are thrown out, producing the double tapping stamping type of gait. Cerebellar ataxias also have a broad-based gait, irregular and unsteady, with or without eyes open, and the child is unable to do tandem walking.

Children with myopathies have a **penguin type of gait** and 'Gower's sign' is positive – the child uses the hands to climb upon himself to stand up from sitting posture. The hypertrophied or bulky calves are seen in these boys, with wasting of the thigh musculature.

Spine

Any head tilt with the chin rotated to the opposite side suggests torticollis or wry neck of the side to which it tilts. In babies one can feel a lump in the sternomastoid which may be the cause and, if not, one should seek other causes such as congenital cervical spinal anomalies. In the older child consider rotary instability of C1–C2 secondary to trauma or parapharyngeal infections (otherwise called Grisel's syndrome); rarely, head tilt can result from ophthalmological causes.

Assess the primary and secondary curves of the spine from the side. From the back the spine should be straight, and any lateral curvature seen is called scoliosis (see Chapter 13). Any list of the upper body and flank creases should be sought. Feel the spine for alignment, tenderness or a step at the lower lumbar spine as in spondylolisthesis.

Forward bending will reveal a structural scoliosis with the development of an asymmetrical rib or lumbar hump (Figure 12.6). Postural or non-structural scoliosis does not show this and can be caused by leg length discrepancy or pain from nerve root entrapment. Scoliosis resulting from leg length inequality can be corrected by using appropriate blocks and making the pelvis level. Structural scoliosis should be assessed for the type of curve and the level of the curve. The usual curve patterns of single right thoracic, single left thoracolumbar or lumbar are those generally seen in adolescent idiopathic scoliosis.

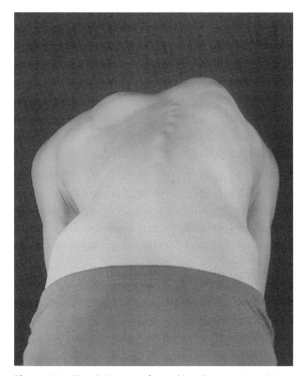

Figure 12.6 The rib hump on forward bending in structural scoliosis.

The flexibility of the curve should then be assessed by side bending and whether part of the curve is correctable can be determined. Decompensation signs of the curve should be assessed by using the plumbline as well as looking at the gait and assessing the secondary curves.

The range of motion of the spine is measured in flexion, extension, lateral flexion and rotation. The latter should be either sitting or by holding the pelvis when standing. Assess true spinal movement in forward flexion, for the hips could compensate. Straight leg raising test, passive and active, should be performed, and this could be restricted because of nerve root irritation as in acute disc protrusion. Tight hamstrings with increased popliteal angles could be a feature of spondylolysis with low back pain, especially in a sporty teenager.

One should be able to assess whether pelvic obliquity influences the spine, or vice versa. This is

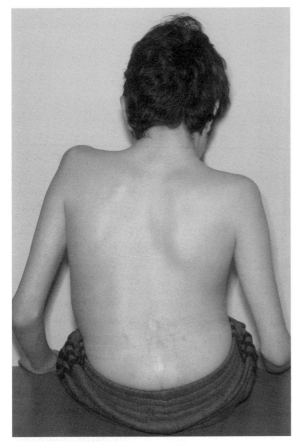

Figure 12.7 Examining sitting to identify any intrapelvic cause of obliquity producing scoliosis.

discussed in the spinal chapter, as suprapelvic, intrapelvic and infrapelvic types, with intrapelvic causes being assessed by revealing hip deformities or by sitting to identify any true hypoplasia of the hemipelvis (Figure 12.7).

Lower limbs

Standing examination includes the Trendelenburg test and the block test for limb length inequality.

Trendelenburg test

Failure of the abductor mechanism, producing a positive Trendelenburg test, is due to instability at the fulcrum in DDH; also, failure of the lever arm, as seen in a short or varus femoral neck, or pseudoarthrosis and failure of the power arm from a neurological cause for weakness of the abductors can result. A positive test is also seen in severe genu varum. A delayed Trendelenburg test assesses abductor fatigue on loading with time and is positive in acetabular dysplasia and coxa vara.

The Trendelenburg test is performed by asking the child to stand on each leg with both hips in extension and the non-weightbearing knee flexed. Normally, standing on the unaffected side elevates the pelvis on the opposite side (Figure 12.8a). A positive test is when the opposite side of the pelvis drops, indicating failure of the abductor mechanism (Figure 12.8b). The delayed Trendelenburg test is to make the child stand for 30 seconds to assess the abductor fatigue. When any associated leg length discrepancy is present, levelling the pelvis with blocks prior to performing the Trendelenburg is advisable lest it produces a false positive result.

Limb length discrepancy

Limb length discrepancy is assessed by the block test (Figure 12.9). Blocks are of different sizes and the child is made to stand with hips and knees extended and feet together with the shorter side on the blocks. The level of the posterior superior iliac spine (PSIS), the highest point of the iliac crests and the ASIS can all be used as landmarks. Examination from the back is more accurate. True shortening can be measured this way only if there is no fixed flexion deformity (FFD) at the hip or the knee. If present, the child should be measured in the supine position, placing the normal leg in the same position as the affected side. The same rule holds good if associated

(a)

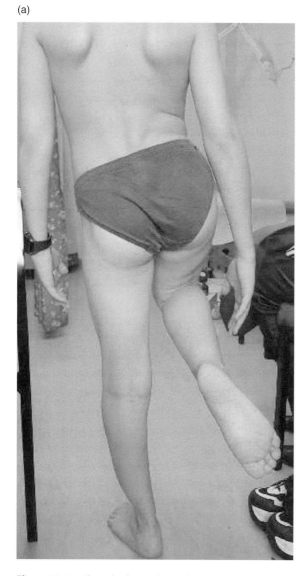

(b)

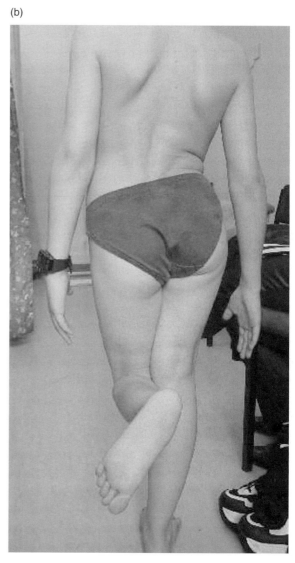

Figure 12.8 a The pelvis being elevated when standing on the unaffected or normal side. **b** The positive Trendelenburg test resulting from Tom Smith arthritis of infancy.

adduction or abduction hip contractures are present. Adduction contracture produces apparent shortening of the limb and abduction contracture makes the leg appear longer.

To determine whether shortening is above or below the knee, the Galeazzi test is performed with the child lying supine and flexing both the knees at a right angle and the heels together. The mismatch in the knee heights when seen from the side and from the end of the bed will suggest whether the

discrepancy is in the femur or tibia (Figure 12.10). Bryant's test can then be used to reveal whether a femoral shortening, if present, is supratrochanteric or infratrochanteric by palpating the relative positions of the tips of the trochanters and ASIS on either side using the thumbs on the ASIS, the middle finger on the tip of the greater trochanter and the index finger perpendicular to the couch. The difference in height between the fingers reveals supratrochanteric shortening.

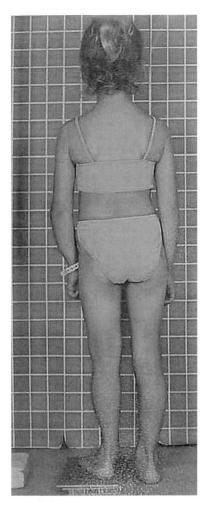

Figure 12.9 The block test to equalize limb lengths.

Rotational profile

The foot and patellar progression angles seen on visual gait analysis will suggest intoeing or outtoeing, but not necessarily identify the segment for the cause. Remember that muscular forces can also influence this, especially in a spastic gait. Prone examination is the best way to determine the site for the torsional anomalies. With the child prone and flexed at the knees, the feet can be assessed for metatarsus varus or other deformities using the heel bisector, or Bleck's line, which normally cuts through the second toe. The thigh–foot angle reflects tibial torsion and is measured by drawing an imaginary line along the long axis of the femur and a line bisecting the foot in its resting position. The normal value is 10–15° of external rotation (Figure 12.11). Alternatively, the transmalleolar axis can be used in the sitting position by comparing the transcondylar axis of the tibia with

(b)

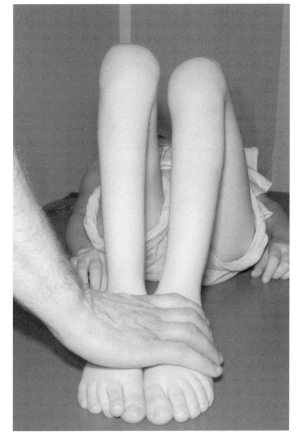

(a)

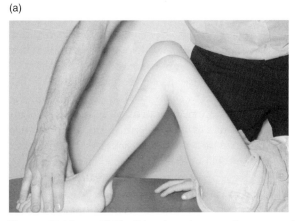

Figures 12.10 a and **b** The Galeazzi test demonstrating asymmetrical knee heights.

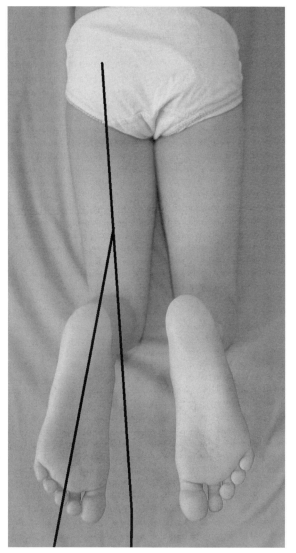

Figure 12.11 The prone examination to assess the thigh–foot angle.

the bimalleolar axis, which is usually about 20° of external rotation.

Next, examine the hip for the range of internal and external rotation and perform the **'Gage test'**, which determines the femoral anteversion. The leg is used as the lever and the axis of the tibia as a reference. The examiner's thumb is placed on the trochanter and the palm of the hand on the buttock. The angle created by the leg to the imaginary vertical line when the greater trochanter becomes most prominent on rotating the limb from maximum internal rotation to maximum external rotation is the angle of

anteversion of the femur. Femoral torsion is described when this is above two standard deviations to the normal. Therefore, there will be excessive internal rotation in femoral torsion and restricted or absent internal rotation in retrotorsion of the hip, as in congenital short femora. Femoral anteversion at birth is about 40°, it is 20° by the age of 9 and reaches the adult value of 12–16° by the age of 16 years.

Hip

General inspection on supine examination is for any scars from previous surgery or sinuses from infection. Any asymmetrical creases, especially at the groin extending to the buttock, may be associated with developmental dysplasia of the hip. The attitude of the limb should be assessed, along with any apparent limb length discrepancy. Any effusion in the joint produces a flexion, abduction and external rotation attitude of the limb as in an irritable hip. The limb appears longer with a fixed abduction deformity and the ipsilateral ASIS is at a lower level. In adduction deformities the limb appears shorter and the ipsilateral ASIS is at a higher level.

Palpate the bony landmarks around the hip for tenderness, including the greater trochanter. Eliciting palpatory findings of the hip joint per se is difficult as it is deeply placed. The femoral head may be palpable in the groin in partially treated DDH or in dysplastic hips; this is the 'lump sign'. The femoral head is made more palpable with the limb held in external rotation. The greater trochanter may be broadened in Perthes' disease.

Before assessing range of motion of the hip joint, concealed deformities need to be revealed. The Thomas test is performed to reveal a FFD at the hip (Figure 12.12). This is concealed by an exaggerated lumbar lordosis. The contralateral hip is flexed to its maximum and held there by the child holding the knee, whilst the examiner confirms flattening of the lumbar lordosis using the palm of his or her hand. The child is then asked to gently extend the other leg. The angle created by the thigh segment with the couch is the angle of the FFD. The range of flexion in this hip is determined and the manoeuvre repeated on the opposite side. The alternative to this test is Staheli's prone hip extension test where the child is stabilized at the bottom of the couch in the prone position with both limbs free and supported; the lordosis is then visually flattened by flexing both hips. The hip is then extended and when

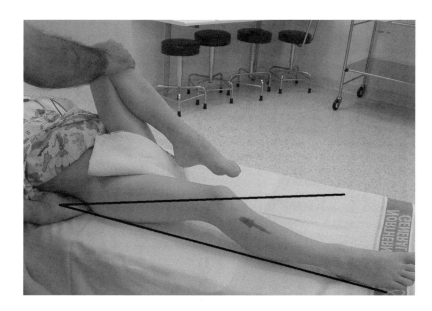

Figure 12.12 The Thomas test to reveal fixed flexion deformity at the hip.

the buttock starts to rise the angle created by the thigh to the lumbosacral spine is the amount of FFD at the hip.

Coronal plane movement is assessed after stabilizing the pelvis and confirming that the pelvis is square. Maximum abduction of the unaffected side is a good method of locking the pelvis. When deformities exist in this plane the pelvis is squared and the further range of motion in that plane is assessed.

Rotation of the hip is best assessed with the hips in extension and the child prone. Rotation with the hip in 90° of flexion can be assessed, but is of less significance.

In irritable hip conditions, the earliest movement lost is adduction in flexion; normally there should be at least 20° in this position.

Telescoping test is positive in late presentation of dislocated hips or old septic arthritis of infancy (Tom Smith arthritis). This is elicited with the hip and knee flexed and, with the pelvis stabilized, the thigh is loaded downwards and released, feeling the femoral head or trochanter moving vertically.

When examining neonates for DDH, the **Ortolani test** is to elicit the sign of entry of the hip from the dislocated position followed by exit to its dislocated position. The test is done with the child relaxed on the couch with one hand stabilizing the pelvis and the other flexing the knee fully and flexing the hip to 90°. The thumb is on the inside with the outer three fingers on the trochanter. As the hip is

abducted, a palpable and audible 'clunk' is a positive test for reduction and when the opposite manoeuvre is performed the clunk of exit is recorded as displacement of the hip. The **Barlow's test** is a provocative test for instability, elicited the same way but demonstrating the clunk of exit from the acetabular rim by gently pushing with the thumb on the adducted hip. Dynamic and static ultrasound examination is the gold standard in assessing instability or dysplasia and monitoring progress of treatment up to the age of 6 months. The later classic signs in DDH are those of asymmetrical thigh folds, limitation of abduction and relative shortening of the femur with the knees in flexion (positive Galeazzi's sign). The Ortolani and Barlow's tests are not useful after the age of 6 months. A plain AP radiograph of the hips after the age of 6 months can be used to diagnose DDH.

Children with Perthes' disease lose abduction in flexion quite early. They also show features of irritability at the hip and gradually also lack internal rotation. When the hip is flexed the knee deviates towards the ipsilateral shoulder. This clinical sign suggests early femoral head deformity. Spasm can produce deformities at the hip and if complicated with chondrolysis can become fixed. Serial AP radiographs and frog leg lateral views will show the different evolutionary stages in the process of healing, from avascular necrosis with the crescent sign, stage of fragmentation or revascularization and healing.

Children with a slipped capital femoral epiphysis have decreased abduction, internal rotation and flexion, whereas they gain adduction, external rotation and extension. Flexing the hip causes the knee to deviate towards the ipsilateral shoulder, as in Perthes' disease. The presence of a FFD as well suggests that the hip is developing chondrolysis. An outtoeing gait is one presentation, especially in chronic slips. A frog leg lateral view of the hips will demonstrate the extent of the slip and also show the early slip, which could be missed in the AP film. The percentage of slip can also be measured on this view.

Knee

Inspect the knee for any swelling. Fullness of the parapatellar fossae suggests a small effusion and a horseshoe swelling of the suprapatellar fossa larger effusions. Generalized swelling is seen in inflammatory synovitis. Localized swellings could result from bursae or bony lumps such as the tibial tuberosity in Osgood–Schlatter's disease. Any colour change with redness and signs of inflammation should be noted. The semimembranous bursa is commonly seen on the posteromedial aspect of the knee. Coronal plane deformities of genu valgum or genu varum should be assessed standing. Up to the age of 2 years, a moderate degree of genu varum is normal. This then develops into excessive valgus by the age of 3 and normalizes to about 7° of valgus by the age of 5–7 years. Pathological causes include the following:

- **Genu varum**: rickets, osteogenesis imperfecta, osteochondromas, achondroplasia, trauma, Blount's disease.
- **Genu valgum**: osteochondromas, renal osteodystrophy, trauma.

The knee is palpated to elicit tenderness at the joint lines for the menisci and bony landmarks (e.g. tibial tuberosity) as well as the patellar undersurface for chondromalacia. For smaller effusions, the bulge test can elicit fluid in the joint and for moderate effusions the patellar tap can be done after squeezing the suprapatellar pouch (Figure 12.13). A tense haemarthrosis does not have a positive patellar tap.

Active range of motion is best elicited before passive movements. Determine whether there is any FFD at the knee as is seen in discoid menisci. Compare the movements of the good knee with the affected one, both in flexion and extension. Hyperextension at the knee is recorded, as well as

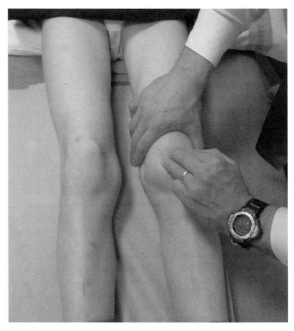

Figure 12.13 Demonstration of the patellar tap.

symmetry and any associated features of benign hypermobility.

Patellar position, whether high (alta) or low (baja), is noted. Patellar tracking in the sitting position with the legs free can demonstrate lateral squinting and tilting, habitual dislocation or subluxation. The patellar apprehension test is elicited by attempting to push the patella laterally in an extended position and then flexing the knee. The child will resist this movement because of discomfort and apprehension if instability exists. Patellofemoral crepitus can be elicited on moving the knee and applying patellofemoral compression against the femoral trochlea. Ligamentous stability should be tested next.

Lachman's test with the knee in 20° of flexion determines abnormal movement in the anteroposterior plane and assesses anterior cruciate deficiency as seen in congenital short femur, or longitudinal deficiencies of the lower limbs as well as in the older child who sustains a tear of the anterior cruciate ligament. Posterior sag of the knee can be assessed with the knee held at a right angle to the couch, demonstrating posterior cruciate deficiency as in some longitudinal congenital deficiencies such as proximal femoral focal deficiency (PFFD) or fibular hemimelia. The latter sign is best investigated first, prior to any other signs for cruciate deficiencies. The collateral ligaments are tested with the knee in extension and in 30° of flexion with varus and valgus force. Ligamentous laxity is associated with many skeletal dysplasias and therefore needs to be recorded.

Foot and ankle

Examine the feet standing, walking and at rest. On standing the heel is in slight valgus to the long axis of the calf because of subtalar mobility. The arch may be flat (pes planus), normal or high (as in pes cavus). Callosities on the sole of the feet inform about the weightbearing pattern and also the soles of the shoes and their uppers. Neuropathic ulcers may be seen in spina bifida and in sensory neuropathic conditions. Deformities of the toes need to be noted. Curly lesser toes, overriding second toes, overriding fifth toes, hammer and mallet toes are some of the common deformities. Clawing of the toes warrants an examination of the spine to exclude spinal dysraphism, as well as investigations for other conditions such as hereditary sensorimotor neuropathies or Friedreich's ataxia. Metatarsus adductus or varus may be noted and could be part of a serpentine or skew foot or a residual clubfoot deformity.

The foot should be palpated over all bony landmarks. Tenderness over the calcaneum could reflect calcaneal apophysitis (Sever's disease). Tenderness around the second metatarsophalangeal (MTP) joint might reflect Freiberg's disease. When assessing mobility of the foot, deformities need to be noted. Ankle range of motion in plantarflexion and dorsiflexion, subtalar movement in eversion and inversion and midfoot movement in all planes needs to be recorded. Any deformity should be assessed as being fixed or correctable, partially or completely. Reduced subtalar movement as in spasmodic peroneal flat foot is seen in tarsal coalitions in adolescents and subtalar irritability is seen in seronegative inflammatory conditions.

Flat feet are associated with dropped medial longitudinal arches on standing and valgus heels. When the child is made to stand on tip toes they recreate the arch and the heel goes into neutral or varus when there is no underlying abnormality. Similar reconstitution of flexible flat feet can be seen on dorsiflexing the big toe and on standing with external rotation of the tibia; this is otherwise described as the 'Jack test'. Flexible flat feet with tight heel cords need to be identified, as they require treatment. Rigid flat feet

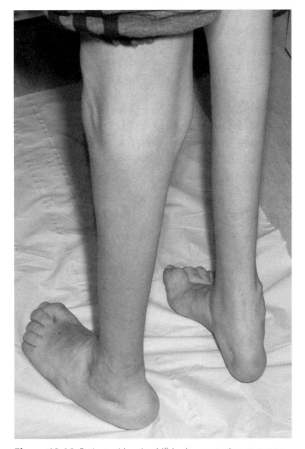

Figure 12.14 Patient with spina bifida demonstrating cavovarus feet and significant wasting of the muscles of the leg.

can be either of the type seen in spasmodic peroneal flat feet of any cause or the rockerbottom type seen in congenital vertical talus or in association with other conditions or syndromes such as spina bifida and arthrogryposis multiplex congenita.

Pes cavus can result from plantaris deformities of the forefoot, equinocavus or in association with calcaneocavus. Remember to look for a neurological cause in patients presenting with a pes cavus (Figure 12.14).

Fixed pronation deformities of the forefoot seen in peroneal muscular atrophy can produce a varus posture of the heel on standing. This may be fully correctable. The Coleman block test can be used to elicit this. The child is asked to stand on a block, which supports the heel and lateral border of the foot, allowing the first metatarsal to drop. The heel should correct to a neutral or valgus position if the hindfoot deformity is mobile, suggesting that the heel varus is due to a fixed pronation deformity of the forefoot.

Examination of the muscles around the foot and ankle is important, and muscle strength should be graded as per MRC grading. Foot deformities can have varying aetiologies, and may be structural as in congenital talipes equinovarus (CTEV), muscular as in Duchenne muscular dystrophy, peripheral nerve disorders as in peroneal muscular atrophy, lower nerve roots as in spinal dysraphism or caused by upper motor neuron disorders, as in cerebral palsy.

Upper limbs
Shoulder

Observe the contour of the shoulder from the front, back and side. A high scapula, as in Sprengel's shoulder, can be seen even from the front. The scapula may be hypoplastic and wider sideways. This could be in association with Klippel–Feil syndrome, with shortening and webbing of the neck and a low posterior hairline. Webbing of the neck may also be seen in Turner's syndrome. Abnormalities of the axillary pectoral folds could be because of absence of the sternal part of the pectoralis major, as in Poland's syndrome. Children with hereditary multiple exostoses often have lumps around the shoulder. Unilateral winging of the scapula can be seen in Parsonage–Turner syndrome and, if bilateral in teenagers, could be an early presentation of facioscapulohumeral or scapuloperoneal dystrophies.

Palpation of the shoulder joint and upper humerus should be performed to elicit tenderness and lumps. Absent clavicles may be seen in cleidocranial dysostosis and defects of the clavicle may be palpable in pseudoarthroses of the clavicle, especially on the right.

Assess the range of motion of the shoulder joint, active first and then passive. The glenohumeral movement is examined by stabilizing the scapula and then the scapulothoracic movements without any restriction of the scapula. Children can be asked to clap their hands in forward flexion or over their heads if not cooperative.

Stability of the shoulder is assessed next by stressing the humeral head forwards and backwards and by the sulcus test by pulling on the arm downwards. Multidirectional instability can be demonstrated in the atraumatic groups with bilateral signs and in

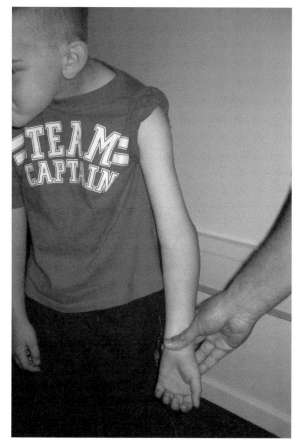

Figure 12.15 Demonstrating cubitus varus after malunion of a supracondylar fracture.

association with ligamentous laxity. The apprehension test for anterior shoulder instability is performed by attempting to abduct and externally rotate the shoulder. The child resists in a positive test. Quite often the child can demonstrate the clunk or instability of the shoulder themselves. It is worth getting the child to elicit this to see the shoulder action and the direction of instability.

Elbow

The elbow is a relatively easy joint to examine in a child. Swelling and deformities are well seen. In full extension the carrying angle can be assessed and is normally 10–15° (more in females). Comparison of the unaffected side gives quantification of any deformity. A reduced carrying angle or cubitus varus is seen in malunited supracondylar fractures (Figure 12.15) and, when severe, produces the

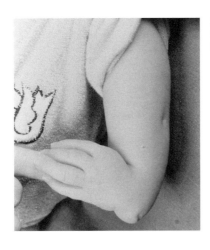

Figure 12.16
Radial club hand
with absent thumb.

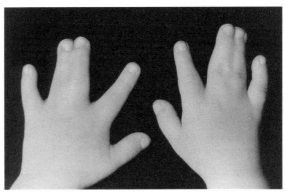

Figure 12.17 Bilateral complete simple syndactyly of both third web spaces.

gunstock deformity, which looks quite unusual when seen from the back or when the child walks. An increased carrying angle is noted in Turner's syndrome.

Palpation of bony landmarks around the elbow is undertaken in a fixed manner. The normal triangular relationship of the epicondyles and tip of the olecranon with the elbow in flexion and the linear relationship with the elbow in extension give clues to assess malunion of the distal humerus. Palpation of the radial head and the assessment of rotation of the forearm may reveal abnormalities of the relationship of the radial head with the capitellum, as in missed Monteggia fractures or congenital dislocation.

Movements of the elbow joint should be recorded and compared to the normal side. Hyperextension can be noted in association with laxity or in malunited supracondylar fractures. With the elbow in flexion at right angles, forearm rotation is assessed. This might be restricted or completely absent in radioulnar synostoses. Examination of shoulder rotation can be used to evaluate varus malunion in supracondylar fractures which results in increased shoulder internal rotation and is best assessed with the child bent forwards and comparing internal rotation from the back (see also Chapter 3, Yamamoto's test).

Wrist and hand

Radial club hand may be mild or severe depending on the state of the radius, which can range from mild hypoplasia to complete absence (Figure 12.16). The condition usually arises sporadically but may be associated with a number of syndromes; for example,

TAR syndrome (thrombocytopenia with absent radii, which is always bilateral), Fanconi anaemia (aplastic anaemia), Holt–Oram syndrome (heart anomalies) and VACTERL (also known as VATER and includes vertebral, anal, cardiac, tracheo-oesophageal, renal and limb defects).

The wrist can be assessed for swellings such as ganglia, classically on the dorsum or the radiovolar aspect. Prominence of the lower end of the ulna with radial and volar deviation of the wrist is seen in a Madelung deformity, and may be bilateral in the familial condition or unilateral if acquired, as in post-traumatic physeal arrest of the distal radius. The wrist can be easily assessed for tenderness, swellings, synovial thickening and any increase in warmth. Movements are assessed and also ligamentous laxity, as seen with hypermobility when the thumb is able to approximate the volar aspect of the wrist.

Generalized systemic disorders can be detected by clubbing or cyanosis of the fingers. Common finger deformities include:

- Kirner deformity – apex dorsal and ulnar curvature of distal phalanx, usually of the little finger
- Clinodactyly – curvature of the digit in the radioulnar plane
- Camptodactyly – flexion deformity of proximal interphalangeal (PIP) joint of the little finger
- Syndactyly – soft tissue or bony connections between the fingers (Figure 12.17)
- Polydactyly – duplication of the digit
- Arachnodactyly – 'spider fingers', a condition where the fingers are abnormally long and slender in relation to the palm (Marfan's syndrome).

Finger movements are also a good indication of ligamentous laxity, with hyperextension at the MCP joints. Joint ranges need to be assessed. Neurological examination is important in post-traumatic sequelae when associated with neurovascular injuries. Abnormalities of sensation may be difficult to assess in the younger child. The sweat pattern of the hand can be examined; if lacking, this is an indication of sensory loss. Examining for individual peripheral nerves and documentation of recovery pattern helps in the follow-up. Any ischaemic sequelae of compartment syndrome need to be identified and differentiated from neurological injury. Asking the child to spread the fingers and demonstrate a 'five', adduct the fingers with the thumb in hand to show a 'four', making a fist and showing the letter 'O' with the thumb and index finger reliably assesses the motor supply of the hand. Strength can be assessed by asking the child to grasp your hand. Test also the pinch and the hook functions.

Neuromuscular examination

Cerebral palsy

The sequence of examination should be in one's own style and has to be modified depending on the age of the child, and whether they can stand and walk or not. To start, children younger than 5 years of age can be examined on their mother's lap. The child who can stand and walk can be assessed standing followed by observational gait analysis, sitting and then supine. The child who cannot walk should be first assessed in the wheelchair followed by sitting and finally supine. Brief upper limb examination, head and neck control and associated defects need to be assessed. Look for athetoid movements or any abnormal dystonic posturing or other abnormal involuntary movements.

Lower limb assessment: range of movements should be recorded methodically and muscle testing carried out as per MRC grading if possible. Leg lengths should be measured with the patient supine, with appropriate positioning depending on pelvic obliquity and contractures. Measurement of the true leg length is important in these children.

Hip: the Thomas test is used to elicit the FFD at each hip and further range of motion is measured. Staheli's prone hip extension test is a worthwhile alternative test as it is more accurate in children with

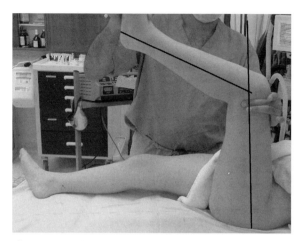

Figure 12.18 The popliteal angle used to assess tight hamstrings.

cerebral palsy. In the same position, hip rotations can also be assessed. The Gage test will determine the angle of femoral anteversion, and femoral torsion is commonly associated with this neuromuscular condition. The prone rectus femoris test demonstrates a tight rectus when the buttock elevates as the knee is rapidly flexed. Hip abduction and adduction should be examined with the hips in extension and in flexion (see Chapter 8).

Knee: spasticity and contracture of the hamstrings can be reliably measured by straight leg raising and assessing the popliteal angle. The hip is flexed to 90° and then the knee is extended from the flexed position. The angle created by the front of the leg to the front of the thigh is the popliteal angle (Figure 12.18). Normal values are less than 20°. Any fixed flexion contracture at the knee should be assessed by extending the limb maximally and, if present, will be due to posterior capsular contracture. Quadriceps strength and spasticity can be assessed next. Phelps' gracilis test is done with the patient prone, knees flexed and hips abducted. If the hip adducts on extending the knee, gracilis spasm or contracture are confirmed.

Foot and ankle: the range of motion at the ankle is recorded. The Silfverskiöld test differentiates gastrocnemius contracture from that of the soleus. If dorsiflexion of the foot is greater when the knee is flexed than when it is extended, then the gastrocnemius is implicated as the main site of contracture. If there is no change, then contracture of both muscles is present. Varus of the foot could be due to a spastic tibialis posterior muscle at the hindfoot or

(a)

(b)

(c)

(d)

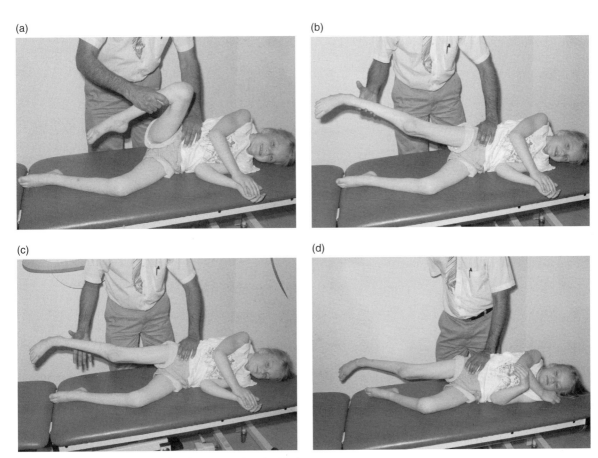

Figure 12.19 The serial sequence for Ober's test as described in the text.

the tibialis anterior at the midfoot or both. It could be a dynamic deformity that is more appreciable when the child walks or a fixed deformity. Tibial torsion needs to be assessed in the sitting position using imaginary lines between the proximal condyles and the distal transmalleolar axis. Alternatively, on prone examination the thigh–foot angle gives an accurate clinical measurement of tibial torsion.

Other paralytic conditions

Knowledge of examining individual muscle groups and for nerve roots is essential in assessing children with paralytic conditions such as poliomyelitis or spina bifida disorders. Sensory dermatomal distribution and knowledge of autonomic systems supplying the bowel and bladder is essential.

Ober's test is used to assess the tightness of the iliotibial band and any abduction contracture at the hip. The test is performed by asking the child to lie on

the side opposite to that being tested. The uninvolved hip and knee are maximally flexed to flatten the lumbar spine. The hip to be tested is flexed to 90° with the knee flexed and then fully abducted. The hip is then brought into full hyperextension and allowed to adduct maximally with a controlled drop. A positive Ober's test is when the limb tends to remain in abduction or has a delayed drop, suggesting tightness of the iliotibial band when it is in maximum stretch (Figure 12.19). The angle that the thigh makes with a horizontal line parallel to the table is the degree of contracture at the hip. When tight, the iliotibial band produces deformities at the knee of flexion, external rotation and valgus, otherwise called the 'triple deformity' (Figure 12.20). Gradual posterior subluxation and secondary deformities of equinus at the ankle, pelvic obliquity, scoliosis and limb length discrepancy may develop; these are classically seen in residual paralysis after poliomyelitis and transverse myelitis.

(a)

(b)

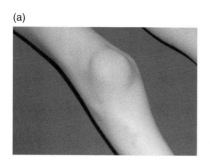

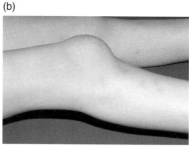

Figure 12.20 The triple deformity of the knee seen in the presence of a tight iliotibial band (flexion, valgus and external rotation).

Summary

Summary of orthopaedic examination in children
There are certain differences in the way that the candidate should approach the child in the exam as opposed to the adult. <ul><li>Remember to communicate with the child as well as the parent</li><li>Examination of the small child does not necessarily need to be on the couch. It can be on the parent's lap or even the floor</li><li>Respect the child's modesty and undress in stages if necessary.</li></ul>

Before examining a paediatric case for abnormalities, it is important to know the variations within normal development.

Developmental milestones

3 months Lifts head when prone
9–12 months Pulls self to stand
15 months Walks unsupported
2 years Runs
3 years Jumps
5 years Hops
6 years Skips

Normal variants

Hip anteversion: 40° at birth; 20° at 9 years; 15° at skeletal maturity.
Knees: 10–15° varus at birth; straight at 18 months; 10–15° valgus at 3 years; 7° valgus from 7 years onwards.
Feet: feet flat at birth; medial arch develops by 6 years.
Lower limb rotational profile (thigh–foot angle): –7° at birth; +7° at 5 years; +10–15° at 10 years onwards.

Based on what observations are made the subsequent examination is tailored

Assessment of rotational profile
Step 1 Walk the patient <ul><li>Foot progression angle</li><li>Patellar progression angle</li></ul>
Step 2 Sit the patient <ul><li>Check transmalleolar axis. This confirms tibial torsion. Normally fibula 20° posterior to medial malleolus. In internal tibial torsion the fibula may be at the same level or in front</li></ul>
Step 3 Lie patient supine (or whilst sitting) <ul><li>Check for metatarsus adductus</li></ul>
Step 4 Lie patient prone <ul><li>Thigh–foot angle. Measure tibial torsion (normal = 10–15° external)</li></ul>
Step 5 Assess external and internal rotation <ul><li>Increased internal rotation with increased femoral anteversion</li><li>Gage's test.</li></ul>

Assessment of a leg length discrepancy
Step 1 Stand patient and look <ul><li>May be standing with pelvic tilt</li><li>FFD of hip or knee</li><li>Expose spine and look for scoliosis.</li></ul>

Step 2
Walk patient

- May see short leg gait.

Step 3
Trendelenburg test

- Shortening of neck results in positive test.

Step 4
Lie patient down

- Square pelvis. Thomas test and hip range of movement
- Tape measure test for true shortening: ASIS to medial malleolus.

If there is a difference then proceed to next steps.

Step 5
Galeazzi's test

- Is shortening above or below knee?

Child supine. Flex both knees to 90° with heels together. Look from side and front to decide if shortening in femur or tibia.
If shortening in the femoral side, then is it above or below the greater trochanter?

Step 6
- Use Bryant's triangle: from the ASIS draw a line downwards. Measure the distance from this line to the tip of the greater trochanter. Compare the two sides.
- Also can use Nelaton's line: draw a line from the ASIS to the ischial tuberosity. The greater trochanter should be on or just below this line.

Step 7
Block test

- The block test is performed by asking the patient to stand on blocks of increasing heights until the pelvis is level and the patient verbally confirms this. It is the most sensitive test of leg length measurement because the tape measure test does not take into consideration shortening arising from below the medial malleolus.

Further reading

Apley AG, Solomon L. *Apley's System of Orthopaedics and Fractures*, 7th edition. Oxford: Butterworth–Heinemann, 1993.

Benson MKD, Fixsen JA, Macnicol MF. *Children's Orthopaedics and Fractures*. London: Churchill Livingstone, 1994.

Bleck EE. *Orthopaedic Management in Cerebral Palsy, Clinics in Developmental Medicine no. 99/100*. Philadelphia: MacKeith Press, 1987.

Broughton NS. *Paediatric Orthopaedics*. Philadelphia: WB Saunders, 1996.

Gage JR. *Gait Analysis in Cerebral Palsy, Clinics in Developmental Medicine no. 121*. Oxford: MacKeith Press, 1991.

Herring JA. *Tachdjian's Pediatric Orthopaedics*, 4th edition. Philadelphia: WB Saunders, 2008.

Sivananthan S, Sherry E, Warnke P, Miller MD. *Mercer's Textbook of Orthopaedics and Trauma*, 10th edition. London: Hodder Arnold, 2012.

Tachdjian MO. *Pediatric Orthopedics*. Philadelphia: WB Saunders, 1990.

Chapter 13

Examination of the spine in childhood

Ashley Cole and Peter Millner

Introduction

The spectrum of conditions of the spine in children includes spinal infection, trauma, tumours, spondylolysis and spondylolisthesis, the adolescent disc syndrome, as well as spinal deformities such as scoliosis.

The clinician should be alerted to the quality and site of any painful spinal symptoms, in terms of whether or not it is activity-related and if there is any neuropathic pain. Worrying symptoms include night pain causing disturbed sleep, unremitting pain requiring regular analgesia and pain interfering with enjoyable activities. The younger the patient, the more likely it is that any spinal tumour is neoplastic, with 75% of spinal tumours in the under-6s being malignant, contrasting with less than 33% in over-6s who have spinal tumours. The benign but painful osteoblastoma and osteoid osteoma occur principally around the thoracolumbar junction and the pain is typically relieved by non-steroidal anti-inflammatory drugs. Although pain is a cardinal feature of spinal malignancy, present in 46–83% of cases, only about one in three cases will present purely with pain and two-thirds will present with neurological problems, such as radicular pain, muscle wasting and weakness and/or a limp. Most children with an underlying neurological or neuromuscular condition will already have a diagnosis, and a previously fit and healthy child who develops new weakness and/or a limp should be suspected of having a spinal tumour until proven otherwise.

The classical triad of fever, spinal pain and spinal tenderness is said to be pathognomonic of spinal infection, but these symptoms are not always all present together at the outset and may be insidious in development, resulting often in a late diagnosis of spinal infection. Constitutional symptoms, such as malaise, fever and weight loss, should suggest spinal infection and sometimes tumour.

Caution should be exercised when dealing with the teenage male with a painful, stiff, progressive, left thoracic scoliosis, particularly when associated with features such as headache or asymmetric abdominal reflexes. A syrinx may be present that can be malignant in origin.

There are a number of different paediatric spinal conditions that require different approaches to both the history-taking and examination. This chapter covers the following three conditions:

1. Scoliosis.
2. Kyphosis/lordosis.
3. Back pain/spondylosis/spondylolisthesis/radicular pain.

Scoliosis

History

Patients with no cause for their scoliosis (idiopathic) are divided into two main groups dependent on age: early-onset scoliosis, with development of deformity before the age of 5 years, and late-onset scoliosis, where the deformity develops after the age of 5 years, often coming to clinical attention in adolescence. Respiratory symptoms are more likely to be associated with early-onset scoliosis, reflecting hypoplasia of the pulmonary vascular and alveolar tree secondary to associated chest wall deformity during and beyond maximal growth and development of the heart and lungs.

The problem: the history should document when and by whom the deformity was first noticed, whether this was some time ago and whether there is a

Examination Techniques in Orthopaedics, Second Edition, ed. Nick Harris and Fazal Ali. Published by Cambridge University Press. © Cambridge University Press 2014.

perception of deformity progression. What was noticed and whether this is of concern to the patient is obviously of key importance in adolescent idiopathic scoliosis (AIS), where the main indication for surgery is to improve trunk cosmesis. Any impact of the spinal deformity at school should be evaluated, as bullying can occur. In wheelchair-bound patients, the first problem noticed by the patient/parents/carers is usually difficulty with sitting balance, especially in those with good upper limb function and cognitive skills. Pressure area problems and particularly hygiene in the skin crease on the concavity of the curve is usually a late feature.

The cause: in apparently fit and healthy children, pain may indicate a cause such as tumour and especially osteoid osteoma, where patients classically have night pain. However, some pain is common in this group and is usually around the area of the curve or in the low back. Worrying features of the pain that may indicate a more sinister cause are:

- Night pain causing difficulty sleeping
- Pain requiring regular analgesia
- Pain causing the patient to be unable to do activities they enjoy
- Any upper or lower limb neurological symptoms.

Fit and healthy children presenting with scoliosis may be a first presentation of:

- Neurofibromatosis, so any family history of neurofibromatosis, skin lesions or birth marks are relevant and can be evaluated on examination, including looking for axillary freckling
- Marfan's syndrome, so any history of eye or cardiac problems and a very tall, slim patient may suggest this diagnosis and prompt looking for a high-arch palate, heart murmur and abnormally long fingers (arachnodactyly) on examination
- Spinal dysraphism, so any upper or lower limb neurological symptoms, bladder or bowel dysfunction or feet abnormalities (pes cavus/toe clawing) should be noted and evaluated on examination.

It is important to elicit any family history of scoliosis and particularly any family history of other diseases as this may suggest the diagnosis of a syndrome or neuromuscular diagnosis. A patient with idiopathic scoliosis has a 20% chance of having a first-degree relative with the same condition, while some conditions associated with spinal deformity are autosomal dominant and therefore carry a 50% risk of transmission from parent to offspring. Many syndromes are associated with scoliosis and sometimes this can be a first presentation; referral for genetic evaluation may be appropriate if there is any suspicion.

Growth, and particularly rapid growth velocity, increases the risk of curve progression, with the other big risk factor for progression being the size of the curve. Infants grow most rapidly between birth and 5 years old, although most patients with infantile idiopathic scoliosis will resolve (80%). There is then a small juvenile growth spurt at about 7–8 years of age. In girls, the adolescent growth spurt normally starts between 11 and 12 years of age, reaching peak growth velocity approximately 6 months before menarche (average age 13.1 years in the UK). Girls will then continue to grow at a reducing growth velocity for 2–2.5 years after menarche. The growth velocity chart for boys is similar but takes place 2 years later than for girls and the peak growth velocity is higher. At first presentation menarcheal status and estimation from the parents regarding growth is useful. Height should be measured for comparison at subsequent visits. In wheelchair-bound patients, growth estimations are much less reliable and menarcheal status can be misleading. Growth is often delayed, but care must be taken as some conditions are associated with early growth, e.g. Sotos syndrome.

Examination

The patient must be undressed to expose the lower limbs and trunk but modesty should be respected, particularly in teenage girls, and the examination can be done in stages. It is often best to examine the trunk first followed by a neurological examination. However, the examination should follow the traditional scheme of look, feel, move and special tests.

Look

The trunk should be inspected from front, side and rear.

Sometimes patients with pectus excavatum and carinatum are sent initially to the paediatric spinal surgeon and are associated with conditions known to be associated with scoliosis, e.g. Marfan's syndrome. Any café-au-lait spots, neurofibromas or axillary

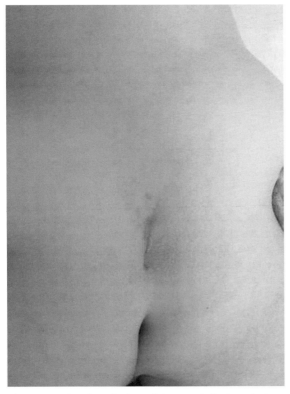

Figure 13.1 Dimple at the base of the spine indicating spinal dysraphism.

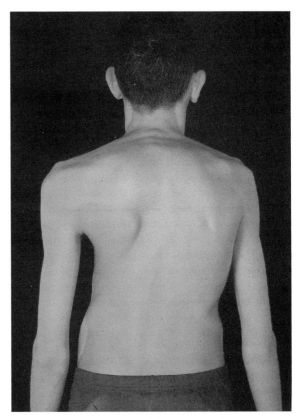

Figure 13.2 Lateral curvature of the spine or scoliosis.

freckling suggestive of neurofibromatosis should be noted. Any scars from previous surgery may be relevant. Signs of spinal dysraphism should be specifically sought, including midline hairy patches or neurofibromas or sacral pits in the natal cleft (Figure 13.1). Klippel–Feil syndrome with a short neck and low hairline may be associated with congenital scoliosis and/or a small high-riding scapula (Sprengel's shoulder).

The asymmetry of the posterior trunk should be assessed in terms of:

- The convex side(s) and anatomical regions of the curve (Figure 13.2)
- Shoulder height asymmetry – high on the right in a right thoracic curve. When the shoulders are level or high on the side opposite the convexity of the main thoracic curve, suspect a compensatory upper thoracic curve
- Rib prominence, which should also be evaluated in a forward bending position by Adam's forward bend test – and can be quantified using a scoliometer (Figure 13.3). This is often large in thoracic scoliosis

- Waist and hip asymmetry (Figure 13.4). In thoracolumbar scoliosis the waist is flattened on the convex side of the curve and the hip is prominent on its concave side
- Frontal plane imbalance assessed by dropping a plumbline from the vertebra prominens which should bisect the natal cleft. In idiopathic scoliosis thoracolumbar curves have the greatest tendency to produce frontal plane imbalance with the head towards the convex side of the curve
- Sagittal shape and balance – kyphosis and lordosis. Idiopathic scoliosis is usually associated with a reduced thoracic kyphosis and this is the hardest plane in which to achieve correction
- Leg length inequality. This can be a cause of postural scoliosis, but scoliosis secondary to leg length inequality can become structural.

Feel

A step in the spinous processes in the lower lumbar spine may suggest a spondylolisthesis associated with AIS. Any abnormal masses should be palpated and,

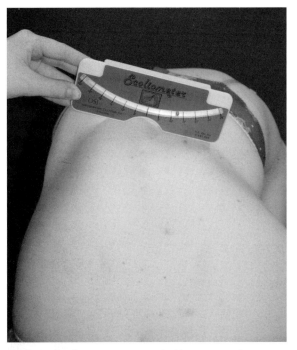

Figure 13.3 Rib prominence quantified by using a scoliometer.

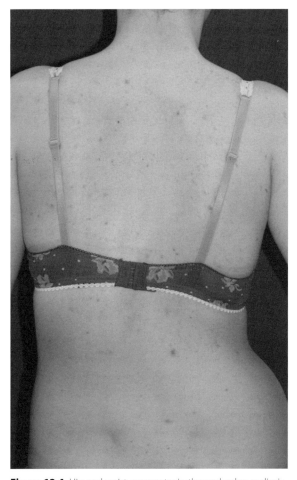

Figure 13.4 Hip and waist asymmetry in thoracolumbar scoliosis.

when there is significant pain, the spine should be palpated and percussed for tenderness.

Move

Spinal movements are rarely helpful, but assessment of flexibility of the curve is very important. In very young patients this can be assessed by suspension. In larger patients, lateral bending or prone stretching can be used. Curve flexibility is crucial in determining timing of spinal surgery where flexible curves can be observed for longer. This is especially important in juvenile idiopathic scoliosis, where delayed surgery may enable a patient to have a fusion rather than more complex growing systems. Care should be taken to observe rotational deformity as this is difficult to correct surgically even in a flexible curve.

Walk

Those patients able to walk should be observed walking with lower limbs exposed. In idiopathic scoliosis this rarely reveals anything unless there is significant pain resulting in a limp or significant leg length inequality. In ambulant patients with syndromes and neuromuscular disease, it is important to assess the effects of the scoliosis on gait and, more importantly, the effects of a potential spinal fusion on gait, especially if the fusion needs to go low into the lumbar spine or even to the pelvis. Patients who rely on increased pelvic rotation during gait may be rendered wheelchair-bound by fusing the spine to the pelvis.

Neurological examination

A full neurological examination is essential in suspected idiopathic scoliosis and this should include assessment of upper and lower limb reflexes, Hoffman's sign (flicking the distal interphalangeal [DIP] joint of the index or middle finger looking for flexion of the thumb interphalangeal [IP] joint), abdominal reflexes, ankle clonus and Babinski reflexes. Reduction in pain and temperature but a normal appreciation of touch indicates the presence of 'suspended' disassociated sensory loss of a syrinx or intramedullary tumour. Examine the feet for pes cavus and claw toes suggestive of an upper motor neuron problem or spinal dysraphism. Any neurological abnormality should prompt a whole spine MRI scan.

Any suggestion of leg length inequality in the standing position should be measured on the couch. Inequality up to 1 cm is considered normal in growing children. Ligamentous laxity should also be assessed, thinking about connective tissue disorders such as Ehlers–Danlos syndrome.

In wheelchair-bound patients the wheelchair should be inspected to see whether there is a moulded seat, bolster support or whether it is patient-controlled, suggesting good cognitive and upper limb function. These patients should be assessed initially sat on the edge of a couch, supported if necessary. The most common curve type is a long C-shaped curve, usually producing marked pelvic obliquity and frontal plane imbalance. There are two causes of pelvic obliquity:

1. Suprapelvic obliquity is caused by a collapsing neuromuscular scoliosis.
2. Infrapelvic obliquity is caused by unequal spasm in the iliopsoas muscles, the only muscles that cross the pelvis from spine to lower extremity. For practical purposes this will only be encountered in cerebral palsy. This may be correctable or fixed; in the latter, when examining leg length inequality in a supine patient the pelvis cannot be put square to the trunk.

To distinguish between these two causes the patient is laid prone at the end of the couch so that the hips can be flexed over the edge of the couch, negating the hip flexion contractures. Abducting and adducting the hips will correct the pelvic obliquity if the cause is infrapelvic whilst there will be no change if the cause is suprapelvic.

The rarer double curve tends to be well balanced in the frontal plane, reducing the indication for surgical treatment. It is also important to assess neck control as patients without neck control are more likely to develop proximal junctional kyphosis after a long instrumentation from the upper thoracic spine to the pelvis. Increased thoracic kyphosis is often associated with neuromuscular disease and often causes seating difficulties resulting from anterior imbalance. An increased lumbar lordosis is often seen in long C-shaped scoliosis in cerebral palsy associated with significant lumbar rotation and this makes any surgical procedure much harder.

Kyphosis/lordosis
History
The history of kyphosis is very similar to that taken for scoliosis:

- Identify the problem
- Assess for an underlying diagnosis
- Assess growth potential
- Evaluate any additional diagnoses that may cause problems with surgery.

These patients will often have back pain in addition to deformity and, as described above, this needs a careful history to try and determine whether there are any sinister features ('red flags'). If the kyphosis has developed quickly and is associated with pain, then a pathological fracture secondary to tumour or infection should be considered. In childhood, a kyphosis secondary to trauma should give an appropriate history of significant trauma.

The two types of idiopathic kyphotic deformity are given the eponymous titles of type 1 and type 2 Scheuermann's disease, depending on the region of the spine affected.

Type 1 Scheuermann's disease (lower thoracic) typically presents in the early to mid teens, whereas type 2 Scheuermann's disease (thoracolumbar) presents in the late teens and early 20s. The presenting features are round back and/or pain over the apex of the deformity. The pain is usually associated with activity and relieved by rest, massage and local heat. Only in the more severe degrees of kyphosis do neurological symptoms ensue, occasionally as thoracic myelopathy. Just like its scoliotic counterpart, management decisions in Scheuermann's disease are determined to a large extent by the patient's perception of their condition, and this should be explored in the consultation.

Other causes of kyphosis include:

- Myelomeningocele producing a significant lumbar kyphosis but often not affecting sitting balance

- Neurofibromatosis: this is often a short angular kyphoscoliosis
- Congenital kyphosis
- Achondroplasia: thoracolumbar kyphosis which usually resolves
- Spondyloepiphyseal dysplasia
- Cervical kyphosis
  - Larsen's syndrome
  - Diastrophic dysplasia
  - Osteogenesis imperfecta.

In patients presenting with kyphosis it is important to ask about neurological symptoms in upper and lower limbs, and particularly about early symptoms of thoracic myelopathy such as an unsteady gait, lower limb sensory changes, bladder and bowel dysfunction and subjective lower limb weakness.

Thoracic lordosis is rare and is usually associated with a syndrome such as Marfan's or Beals. It is an important condition as the narrowed anteroposterior chest diameter can have a significant detrimental effect on respiratory function, which is usually progressive.

Examination

Inspection should evaluate the kyphosis/lordosis. These deformities are almost always rigid except when combined with neuromuscular disease in wheelchair-bound patients. Juvenile idiopathic kyphosis is more common in teenage boys and acne is often present. This should be noted, as it may increase the risk of infection following a surgical procedure and can be improved with a short course of treatment. Posture is very important, as shoulder protraction and a stooped posture can accentuate a thoracic kyphosis significantly and correcting this may eliminate the requirement for surgery. This posture is often adopted in the teenage population affected by juvenile idiopathic scoliosis. Tight localized kyphosis is typical in pathological kyphosis (usually painful), neurofibromatosis and congenital kyphosis. Localized kyphosis has a higher risk of spinal cord compression.

Palpation and movement are not helpful. Gait should be assessed, with a broad-based unsteady gait suggesting myelopathy and spinal cord compression.

A full neurological examination is essential (see above).

Back pain
History

Low back pain in childhood is very common, with an incidence of 37%. Whilst it is less common to find a definite cause for back pain in patients over the age of 10 years and very rare to find a sinister cause, each case should be evaluated in the same way.

In childhood and particularly in teenagers, lumbar disc protrusions do occur and, although they may produce radicular leg pain, they often just give back pain. Radicular pain in childhood is rare and always justifies an MRI scan. If the lumbar spine MRI is normal, then a pelvic MRI should be performed as tumour must be excluded.

A fatigue fracture of the pars interarticularis (spondylolysis) and a forwards slip of one vertebra on the vertebra below (spondylolisthesis) are among the most common causes of childhood and adolescent low back pain. However, spondylolyses are seen in 3% of 3-year-olds, 10% of Caucasian adults and up to 50% of Inuit (Eskimo) Indians. In most adults with the condition, they are an incidental finding with only a weak or no linkage to back pain. Painful symptoms associated with these conditions are often reported by individuals who subject their spines to repetitive extension and twisting: ballet dancers, gymnasts and fast bowlers (cricketers), although in most the symptoms will settle with cessation of the provocative activity. Occasionally, if hypertrophic callus builds up at the site of the spondylolysis, this can irritate the exiting nerve root and cause dermatomal pain or sensory disturbance, but rarely motor dysfunction. As most spondylolyses occur at L5, and most spondylolistheses are of L5 on S1, it is the L5 nerve root that is usually affected.

Thoracic back pain is also common in childhood and may be associated with an increased kyphosis or radiological changes of Scheuermann's disease. Thoracic pain should have a high level of suspicion for sinister pathology and should be investigated with an MRI scan or bone scan for younger patients where the level of suspicion is low.

Rheumatological conditions can present in childhood especially ankylosing spondylitis and juvenile chronic arthritis. The presence of other affected joints or significant early morning spinal stiffness may suggest these diagnoses. There may be a family history of ankylosing spondylitis. SAPHO (synovitis, acne,

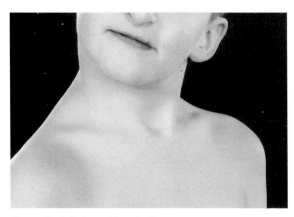

Figure 13.5 Patient with torticollis.

pustulosis [palms and plantar], hyperostosis [sternoclavicular] and osteitis) can present with back pain. The combination of clinical features and anterior vertebral body and endplate erosion suggest this diagnosis.

Neck pain is less common in childhood and should raise suspicion of sinister pathology. Neck clicking is very common and this can be very audible. Imaging investigation does not reveal a cause.

Examination

Gait should be observed as a limp may be present and walking may be obviously painful. This suggests sinister pathology such as infection or tumour. Inspect for any abnormal masses, overall spinal shape and frontal and sagittal plane balance. A scoliosis may be present owing to muscle spasm secondary to a painful intraspinal problem (such as infection, tumour or even prolapsed disc) or a paraspinal focus (such as renal tract pathology). The examination should be used to confirm where the patient experiences the pain to define an anatomical level. Focal pain should be considered more sinister than generalized pain. Tenderness may be elicited on palpation or percussion. Any spinous process step in the low lumbar spine may suggest a spondylolisthesis. Spinal movements in the area of concern should be assessed: flexion, extension and lateral flexion in the lumbar spine; rotation in the thoracic spine and flexion, extension, rotations and lateral flexions in the cervical spine. Loss of movement or pain should raise suspicion.

Passive straight leg raise may be restricted because of tight hamstrings, which are common in rapidly growing children, but may also reflect a spondylolysis or spondylolisthesis. A positive stretch test reproducing radicular leg pain or low back pain may suggest a lumbar disc protrusion.

Neurological examination should be performed, especially looking for problems that are unlikely to have been noted by the patient: extensor hallucis longus weakness suggestive of L5 radiculopathy or weakness on tip toe stance suggestive of S1 radiculopathy, reflex abnormalities, including abdominal reflexes, Hoffman's sign if cervical spine pathology is suspected, Romberg's test, ankle clonus and Babinski reflex.

Torticollis

It is important to establish the length of time a torticollis has been present. Torticollis since birth suggests sternomastoid tightness, especially if there is a history of a sternomastoid lump, which usually disappears by 4 months. This condition resolves with stretching and positioning and is not painful.

Painful or late-onset torticollis should be considered an urgent condition. Atlantoaxial rotatory subluxation is diagnosed with a CT scan rotating the neck to left and right and is often preceded by an upper respiratory tract infection (Grisel's syndrome).

In torticollis, the neck tilts to one side (the side of the torticollis) and rotates to the other (Figure 13.5). It is often difficult to see a tight sternomastoid, but it is always worth checking for scars in the neck and particularly evidence of a previous sternomastoid release (proximally just below the mastoid and distally just above the clavicle). Also seek scars posteriorly that are suggestive of previous surgery to the cervical spine. Palpating the sternomastoid may reveal a tight muscle or sternomastoid swelling in congenital muscular torticollis. The absence of a tight sternomastoid may suggest an alternative cause, such as a structural problem in the upper cervical spine (atlantoaxial rotatory subluxation being the most common) or a posterior fossa tumour. When evaluating movements, it is important to note whether the neck can be tilted to a neutral position or beyond actively and passively, and whether the rotation is correctable.

Summary

Summary of examination of the child with scoliosis

The assessment of the scoliosis patient is very similar to the lumbar spine examination (see Chapter 7) except for a few points mentioned below.

Scoliosis

- Stand and look
- Feel
- Move
- Walk
- Lie the patient down

Complete neurological examination
Provocative tests

Additional points on examination:

1. On looking, **look** for any stigmata for the cause (e.g. neurofibromas, high-arch palate, pes cavus, etc.).
2. When **feeling** you can assess the balance of the spine by using a plumbline.
3. When asking patient to **move**, in forward flexion look for a rib hump (structural scoliosis).
4. When performing the **neurological examination**, include the abdominal reflex, as this is an indicator of thoracic pathology.

Further reading

Akbarnia BA, Yazici M, Thompson GH (eds). *The Growing Spine*. New York: Springer, 2011.

Dickson RA, Millner PA. The child with a painful back. *Curr Orthop* 2000;**14**:369–379.

Index